WITHDRAWN

EL DORADO COUNTY LIBRARY

3 1738 00408 3547

S0-CCX-830

EL DORADO COUNTY FREE LIBRARY
345 FAIR LANE
PLACERVILLE, CALIFORNIA 95667

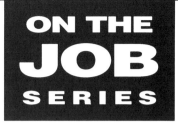

ON THE JOB SERIES

REAL PEOPLE WORKING *in*

HEALTH CARE

Blythe Camenson

Printed on recyclable paper

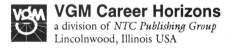

VGM Career Horizons
a division of *NTC Publishing Group*
Lincolnwood, Illinois USA

EL DORADO COUNTY FREE LIBRARY
345 FAIR LANE
PLACERVILLE, CALIFORNIA 95667

Dedication

To my "Little Sister," Shalonda Larkin who, one day, might join the ranks of medical professionals.

Library of Congress Cataloging-in-Publication Data
Camenson, Blythe.
    Real people working in health care / Blythe Camenson.
       p.   cm.—(On the job)
    Includes bibliographical references and index (p.).
    ISBN 0-8442-4725-1. (hbk. : alk. paper).—ISBN 0-8442-4727-8
(pbk. : alk. paper)
    1. Medicine—Vocational guidance.   I. Title.   II. Series.
R690.C36   1997
610.69—dc20   96-266710
                                       CIP

Published by VGM Career Horizons, a division of NTC Publishing Group
4255 West Touhy Avenue
Lincolnwood (Chicago), Illinois 60646-1975, U.S.A.
© 1997 by NTC Publishing Group. All rights reserved.
No part of this book may be reproduced, stored in a retrieval
system, or transmitted in any form or by any means,
electronic, mechanical, photocopying, or otherwise,
without the prior permission of NTC Publishing Group.
Manufactured in the United States of America.

67890 VL 987654321

Contents

Acknowledgments

The author would like to thank the following professionals for providing information about their careers:

- Bobbie Campbell, Sports Medicine Nurse
- Helen Cox, Occupational Therapist
- Sherry Crespo, Physician Assistant
- Laurie DeJong, Physical Therapist
- Dr. Ernest DiGeronimo, Plastic Surgeon
- Fay Dudley, Speech-Language Pathologist
- Eileen Edgecomb, Dental Hygenist
- Emily Friedland, Dietitian
- Deanna Fusco, Medical Secretary
- Dr. Daniel Hurwitz, General Practitioner
- Dr. David Kagan, Dentist
- Dr. Mark Kaufman, Urologist
- Bertha Lovelace, Nurse Anesthetist
- Frank Maluda, Pharmacist
- Tania Maxwell, EMT
- Stephie Morin, Certified Nurse Midwife
- Woody Poitier, Paramedic
- Brad Potts, Nurse Practitioner
- Commander Harry Small, EMS Supervisor
- Dr. Lance Weidenbaum, Veterinarian
- Dr. Ronie Zaruches, Optometrist

About the Author

A full-time writer of career books, Blythe Camenson's main concern is helping job seekers make educated choices. She firmly believes that with enough information, readers can find long-term, satisfying careers. To that end, she researches traditional as well as unusual occupations, talking to a variety of professionals about what their jobs are really like. In all of her books she includes first-hand accounts from people who can reveal what to expect in each occupation, the upsides as well as the down.

Camenson's interests range from history and photography to writing novels. She is also director of Fiction Writer's Connection, a membership organization providing support to new and published writers.

Camenson was educated in Boston, earning her B.A. in English and psychology from the University of Massachusetts and her MEd in counseling from Northeastern University.

In addition to *On the Job: Real People Working in Health Care*, the other books she has written for VGM Career Horizons are:

Career Portraits: Travel

Career Portraits: Writing

Career Portraits: Nursing

Career Portraits: Firefighting

Careers for History Buffs

Careers for Plant Lovers

Careers for Health Nuts

Careers for Mystery Buffs

Great Jobs for Communications Majors

On the Job: Real People Providing Services

Opportunities in Museums

Opportunities in Teaching English to Speakers of Other Languages

How to Use This Book

On the Job: Real People Working in Health Care is part of a series of books designed as companion books to the *Occupational Outlook Handbook*. The *OOH*, as it is commonly called, is a great reference book useful for librarians, guidance and career counselors, as well as job seekers. It provides information on hundreds of careers, focusing on the following subjects:

> Nature of the Work
>
> Working Conditions
>
> Employment
>
> Training, Other Qualifications, and Advancement
>
> Job Outlook
>
> Earnings
>
> Related Occupations
>
> Sources of Additional Information

What the *OOH* doesn't provide is a first-hand look at what any particular job is *really* like. And that's where our *On the Job* series picks up the slack. In addition to providing an overview of each field, training and education requirements, salary expectations, related fields, and sources to pursue for further information, *On the Job* authors have talked to dozens of professionals and experts in the various fields.

These first-hand accounts tell what each job really entails, what the duties are, what the lifestyle is like, what the upsides and downsides are. All of the professionals reveal what drew them to the field and how they got started. And so you can make the best career choice for yourself, each professional offers you some expert advice based on years of personal experience.

Each chapter also lets you see at a glance, with easy to reference symbols, the level of education required and salary range for the featured occupations.

So, how do you use this book? Easy. You don't need to run to the library or buy a copy of the *OOH*. All you have to do is glance through our extensive table of contents, find the fields that interest you, and read what the experts have to say.

Introduction to the Field

The health service industry leads all others as the largest employer in the United States. If you're reading this book, chances are you're already considering a career in this fast-growing and exciting profession. Glancing through the table of contents will give you an idea of all the choices open to you.

But perhaps you're not sure of the working conditions the different fields offer or which area would suit your personality, skills, and lifestyle the most. There are several factors to consider when deciding which sector of health and medicine to pursue. Each field carries with it different levels of responsibility and commitment. To identify occupations that will match your expectations, you need to know what each job entails.

Ask yourself the following questions and make note of your answers. Then, as you go through the following chapters, compare your requirements to the information provided by the professionals interviewed inside. Their comments will help you pinpoint the fields that would interest you, and eliminate those that would clearly be the wrong choice.

- How much patient care do you want to be involved in? Not every field offers the same amount or same type of people contact.

- How strong is your interest in the actual science supporting the different fields? Some occupations require more knowledge and more involvement than others.

- How much time are you willing to commit to training? Some skills can be learned on-the-job or in a year or two of formal training; others can take up to ten years or more.

- How much money are you willing or able to invest in that training, or in possibly starting a private practice? For some fields the outlay can be daunting. New graduates can start out owing many thousands of dollars.

- How much money do you expect to earn after you graduate and after you have a few years' experience under your belt? In general, those areas that pay the most also require the largest investment of time and money.

- Will the actual work offer enough of a challenge? Will it provide you with a sense of accomplishment, or will it become tedious after you've learned the ropes?

- How much independence do you require? Do you want to be your own boss or will you be content as a salaried employee?

- Will you work normal hours? Or will your day start at 5:30 A.M. and not end until 13 or 14 hours later? Can you handle emergency calls in the middle of the night? Do you want your weekends free?

- How much stress can you handle? Would you prefer to avoid work that could be emotional draining?

Knowing what your expectations are, then comparing them to the realities of the work, will help you make informed choices.

Although *On the Job: Real People Working in Health Care* strives to be as comprehensive as possible, not all jobs in this extensive field have been covered or given the same amount of emphasis. If you still have questions after reading this book, there are a number of other avenues to pursue. You can find out more information by contacting the sources listed at the end of each chapter. You can also find professionals on your own to talk to and observe as they go about their work. Any remaining gaps you discover can be filled by referring to the *Occupational Outlook Handbook.*

CHAPTER 1

Medical Doctors

🎓 **EDUCATION**
Post Graduate Required

💲💲💲 **SALARY/EARNINGS**
$75,000+

OVERVIEW

Medical doctors, or physicians as they are also known, examine patients; obtain medical histories; order, perform, and interpret diagnostic tests; and treat injuries, illnesses, and disorders. They also consult with other physicians and, if they are in private practice, take care of the business aspects of running an office.

Training for doctors is long and arduous, and once licensed and in practice the load doesn't decrease. Doctors have irregular schedules, and often work between 50 and 60 hours a week.

JOB SETTINGS

About two out of three doctors have an office-based practice or work in clinics or HMOs; about one-fifth of all doctors are employed by hospitals. Others work for the federal government in veterans' hospitals, or for the Public Health Service in the Department of Health and Human Services.

While traditionally doctors have always been solo players, it is becoming more and more common to see partnerships or group practices. This arrangement allows doctors to be able to afford expensive equipment and enjoy other business advantages.

TRAINING

Most students enter medical school, which takes four years of study, with a bachelor's degree or even higher, then go on to do a residency.

Premedical studies include undergraduate work in biology, physics, and organic and inorganic chemistry.

The first two years of medical school include coursework in anatomy, biochemistry, physiology, microbiology, pathology, medical ethics, and laws governing medicine.

During the last two years, students work under the supervision of experienced physicians learning acute, chronic, preventive, and rehabilitative care. Through rotations in family practice, internal medicine, obstetrics and gynecology, pediatrics, psychiatry, and surgery, med students gain experience working directly with patients, diagnosing and treating illnesses.

After medical school, and after passing an examination given by the National Board of Medical Examiners, almost all new M.D.s go on to do a residency. The residency can take up to seven years depending upon the specialty they are pursuing. A subspecialty might require an additional one to two years of residency. After the residency is completed, doctors sit for a final examination given by The American Board of Medical Specialists. This is required for board certification.

Specialties

There are many areas of medicine in which a doctor can practice. Board certification is required for 23 specialties. They are: allergy and immunology; anesthesiology; colon and rectal surgery; dermatology; emergency medicine; family practice; internal medicine; neurological surgery; nuclear medicine; obstetrics and gynecology; ophthalmology; orthopedic surgery; otolaryngology; pathology; pediatrics; physical medicine and rehabilitation; plastic surgery; preventive medicine; psychiatry and neurology; radiology; surgery; thoracic surgery; and urology.

EARNINGS

Earnings vary according to specialty; the number of years in practice; geographic region; hours worked; and skill, personality, and professional reputation.

According to the AMA (American Medical Association), average salaries after expenses run about $170,000 a year. A recent survey the AMA conducted reveals that general practitioners earn on average $98,000 a year, with income going up with the different specialties. The top of the scale shows radiologists earning $223,000 a year after expenses.

But these are just averages. Some specialties or well-run office practices can pull in $500,000 a year or more. To offset this, it is important to remember that most doctors in private practice outlay a considerable sum of money for equipment and insurance, and most new doctors have astronomical medical school loans to pay off.

RELATED FIELDS

Physicians work to prevent, diagnose, and treat diseases, disorders, and injuries. Professionals in other occupations that require similar kinds of skill and critical judgment include acupuncturists, audiologists, chiropractors, dentists, doctors of osteopathy (D.O.), optometrists, podiatrists, speech pathologists, and veterinarians.

INTERVIEW
Dan Hurwitz
Family Practitioner

Dan Hurwitz became an M.D. in 1974. After three years of postgraduate training in family practice, he set up his own office. Working with him are a nurse practitioner, two medical assistants, and two front office people.

What the Job's Really Like

"Because I can't get all the paperwork done during the day, when I finish the evening hours, instead of staying around in the office dictating, I bring the charts home. A typical day starts with me getting up in the morning around 5:30, quarter to 6, and I'll dictate the remaining charts, for whatever amount of time it takes; it could be half an hour or 45 minutes. Then I'll go to the hospital and make rounds. These are patients who have been hospitalized for medical problems, such as a heart attack, heart failure, pneumonia, severe kidney infection, etc. I would also hospitalize surgical patients. For example, I had an elderly patient who fell down and broke her hip. I hospitalized her and did a consult with the orthopedic surgeon who did the surgery, while I provided all the internal medical care. I'm on staff at two hospitals, but usually my patients are just at one, which makes life a little bit easier. I always try to finish my rounds on time so I can get to the office for my first appointment at nine o'clock.

"I see a range of patients with a range of problems. From chronic illnesses such as hypertension, diabetes, or heart disease to a multitude of acute problems such as upper or lower respiratory problems. Every day, I schedule two complete physical examinations. This is mainly for preventive medicine and because they take a lot more time, I can only do two a day. I schedule one for the first patient in the morning, the other for the first patient in the afternoon.

"The other patients I see are a combination of patients who have been scheduled in advance for follow-up visits for their chronic or acute illnesses and acute patients who called in that day.

"The real benefit to my job, to family practice, is being able to develop a continuing relationship with the patient and the patient's family–meaning I have patients who have been with me as long as I've been in practice. The specialist will often see a patient for a certain problem. For example, I'll send a patient to a vascular surgeon. He'll do the surgery, then kiss him goodbye. Whereas, with my practice, I have a continuing relationship and that's very important and very rewarding to me.

"There are a bunch of negative aspects. Government intervention is one. In days gone by I used to have a lab in my office. It wasn't an extensive lab, but I could do blood counts and urine cultures and a number of other tests on the spot. It was practicing good medicine. A patient would come in to see me with, for example, abdominal pain, and I could see right away if the white blood count was high and if there was a potential problem or need for hospitalization. But now I can't do that, the government won't allow it unless you meet certain stipulations that I don't want to participate in. It's really cut into my practice of medicine.

"And I don't enjoy the copious paperwork I have to deal with. There are also frustrations dealing with patients who have difficulty complying with medical advice. People who keep smoking, people who don't take their medicines appropriately.

"The other consideration is the malpractice problem. It's a very litigious society and everybody is out to lay their suit. So you're constantly making sure that you're dotting that "i" and crossing that "t" and documenting everything you can into the chart. You don't want someone to come back at you one day and try to level a suit at you. That's an unpleasant part of medicine.

"But, the most pleasant part is that I think the practice of medicine is not pure science; it's both art and science. I think in family practice, especially, you get to practice both the art and science of medicine. And that makes life more enjoyable."

How Dan Hurwitz Got Started

"It goes way, way back to a nice Jewish mother who put a lot of emphasis on the professions. That was a major factor as a starting point. I also knew that whatever I ended up doing, I wanted to be independent, to be in charge of my life and not have to answer to anybody. And when I say that, I mean that I have my own practice, I run the office myself, the way I feel it needs to be run. I don't have to worry about having a boss, punching a time card, or being fired at a moment's notice. But things have changed through the years and they've changed tremendously. In the old days you ran a very independent practice, with, but separate from, Medicare and private insurances and you could do as you saw fit. But now we have to jump through many hoops. It is becoming more and more regulated and that's a problem now, and not why I went into medicine.

"Another component of why I chose this profession was that I wanted to be able to work with people, because I feel I have a lot of empathy. And the final component was that the profession is challenging.

"When I started medical school I had wanted to be a pediatrician. I was very interested in working with children. During medical school you rotate through all the different specialties, internal medicine, ob/gyn, surgery, pediatrics, family medicine. And lo and behold I finished the first year and I found out there were big people, too. I discovered I really liked the concept of being able to deal with the entire family, doing family medicine, dealing with the parents, the grandparents, the children.

"I went to college at NYU and graduated in 1970. I went to medical school at the University of Miami and graduated in 1974. Then I did three years of post-graduate training in family practice; the first two years were in Columbus, Ohio, the third year was at Jackson Memorial Hospital in Miami."

Expert Advice

"Getting into medical school is exceedingly difficult. It doesn't really make sense, but with more government regulations and more problems in medicine than ever before, we're getting more applicants than ever before. Probably the most important thing for a student considering a premed course is that the first year in college is most important. Freshman year students are often feeling their oats and enjoying their liberties and might not be studying quite as much as they should. If, by the time the second year rolls around, and they decide they really want to go into medicine, but their first year was not very successful, it can really drag them down. Have fun, enjoy yourself, but really try to concentrate on academics and not get behind the eight ball. Then they have the opportunity to make the decision whether or not to pursue medicine. This is as opposed to blowing that first year and not being able to have the choice. If you start out with a low GPA, it's almost impossible to catch up."

INTERVIEW

Mark Kaufman
Surgeon/Urologist

Mark Kaufman became an M.D. in 1979. With his partner, he operates two offices in Miami, Florida.

What the Job's Really Like

"A urologist is a surgeon who specializes in the surgical diseases of the urinary tract in men and women. I operate on kidneys, ureters, bladders, genitals. My patients are people of all ages with a wide variety of problems ranging from urinary tract infections to cancers of the kidney, prostate–everything–voiding dysfunction, urinary symptoms that are unexplained otherwise, male infertility.

"Urology is unique in the sense that we're half-time in the hospital, half-time in the office. Some specialties, such as general surgery, for example, are mainly hospital-based. They spend most of their time in the hospital and don't usually have an office practice. Some medical doctors rarely go to the hospital or they spend very little time there. I work out of about six different hospitals. I have one partner and we're looking for a third.

"I wake up anywhere from 6:15 to 7:30 and I operate most days. Generally, I do surgeries in the morning, though that can vary. I'll do anywhere from one to three operations in the morning. In between surgery I'll see patients in the hospital who are recovering from surgery. So we run around a lot.

"Occasionally, I'll be called in when someone else is doing surgery, if they're having a problem. And I do a lot of consulting.

"Then I go into the office and I spend a lot of time answering phone calls from other doctors, from patients, from families, home health agencies. And answering the mail, which can hold anything from subpoenas for medical records to lab results. And we get a lot of garbage mail, too. Tons of paperwork. I spend a minimum of two to three hours a day with paperwork alone. Then I'll start off with office hours and see anywhere from 20 to 30 people in an afternoon. How much time I spend with each patient varies. It could be two to five minutes to a half hour.

"While I'm seeing patients, the phone doesn't stop ringing. Between the two offices I have about eight staff people. Most are medical assistants or what we call back room people. They help with procedures I perform in the office. Then we have front desk people, who make appointments, schedule surgeries, all sorts of functions.

"You have all the headaches of running any kind of office, except there are some unique features to it in the sense that there are a lot of legal issues that have to be considered. Medical records are confidential. And you have to monitor your medical records. You have to be careful what goes into a chart and make sure that your staff didn't file a biopsy report showing someone has cancer and you didn't see it. You have to be very meticulous.

"And you have to deal with medical regulations, OSHA, CLIA regulations. Basically, they make your life miserable when you're running a lab in a physician's office.

"Anyone who goes into medicine, you should know that you'll have the government on your shoulder telling you what you can and can't do. It's the most regulated industry in the world, with more watch dog agencies, bureaucrats, third-party payers, attorneys, and insurance companies, waiting for you to make a mistake so they can blame you. It's very high pressured.

"I never have two days that are identical. I finish up at 6 or 6:30 and sometimes I have to go back to the hospital then. And I'm on every other weekend and have to make rounds at the hospitals. It's not too bad with urology, but occasionally we get our share of middle-of-the-night calls. And when you're on call you have to be available. You wear your beeper and carry your cellular phone. It's basically a noose around your neck.

"The upside is that medicine is wonderful, doing surgery is great. There's a certain mystique about it. You're invading someone's body to go in and fix something and it requires certain skills. You have to know when to operate, when not to operate, how to operate, and what operation to do.

"Recently, I operated on a little seven-year-old boy who'd been hit by a car. His kidney was totally shattered, he had broken bones and blood in his abdomen. We saved his life and that's a reward nobody else can get.

"But then, of course, you have to know how to take care of any complications afterwards. I had one guy this week. We did a major operation on him, and for two days his kidneys didn't work for some unexplained reason. They finally kicked in, but needless to say, that's a little extra work and a little extra worry."

How Mark Kaufman Got Started

"My father was a physician and it was basically all I was ever going to do. Doctors were very respected and it was something special. I have a B.S. in general science from Brandeis University in Waltham, Massachusetts. I did four years undergrad, four years of medical school at Washington University, then after medical school, I did a residency for five years. Two of those years were at the medical college in Richmond, Virginia doing general surgery. By then you're an M.D. and you're practicing, but you're in a teaching institution with full-time attending faculty who watch what you're doing and you're still learning. Then I spent three years at Jackson Memorial at the University of Miami in urology.

"I chose urology for a couple of reasons. One, I wanted to do surgery and, in my mind, urology has the best mix of everything. We take care of all ages. We do everything from minor procedures to complex procedures. We have the most variety.

"But the main reason was that I spoke to a lot of surgeons and urology seemed to have the highest degree of satisfaction. We're specialized enough that we're not competing with other surgeons to do what we do, but not so specialized that we get bored doing it.

"And, we, as a specialty, probably have more satisfied patients. If you've had a stroke and you go to a neurologist, for example, there's not a helluva lot they can do. But if you come to me with a kidney stone or urinary tract infection, there's something we can do and there's a very high degree of immediate reward."

Expert Advice

"My advice is don't expect medicine to be what you imagined it to be. Most doctors who started when I did, or even prior to that, are fiercely independent people and don't want to be told what to do. They've been trained to take care of people and to make decisions—not have people who are maybe high school graduates sitting in front of a computer terminal at an insurance company telling you what to do.

"The doctor of the future will, unfortunately, be working for businessmen. And the businessmen will be making the decisions that will impact the patients.

"You have to go into medicine with open eyes. You'll spend a lot of years training and you give up a lot. This is during your younger years, while most people are building equity in their homes and starting businesses. But you won't make any money until you've been in practice five years or so. You spend four years in college, four years in medical school, five years in residency, and five years in practice and it's a long time to wait for the so-called big bucks.

"It's a long road and you have to be very persistent and money shouldn't be the reason you go into this now. You have to make sure it's something you'll really love doing."

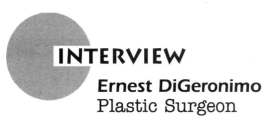

INTERVIEW

Ernest DiGeronimo
Plastic Surgeon

Ernest DiGeronimo sees about 30 patients a day. He has 4,000 square feet of office space with two operating rooms. He employs a certified registered nurse practitioner, an office administrator, three secretaries/receptionists, an insurance clerk, a nurse anesthetist, and a medical assistant who organizes the operating rooms and assists him in surgery.

What the Job's Really Like

"When I was in training, I worked with every aspect of plastic and reconstructive surgery. Birth defects, patients who've had accidents or amputations, cancer patients. But in private practice, those traumatic cases would not go to you, they'd go to an emergency room. Or you'd have to work in a university hospital setting to see them.

"I deal with elective, cosmetic surgery such as face lifts; eye lifts; nose refinements; breast augmentations, reductions, and lifts; abdominoplasty–tummy tucks; and also liposuction or liposculpturing.

"My work is better than I ever imagined it would be starting out. You get people who want something and you're able to deliver it and deliver it well. It fulfills me. A hobby of mine is art and antiques and I actually restore antiques. I kind of do the same thing in my work. Take people and restore them.

"The downsides are that you're working with people who already look pretty darn good and want that extra mile or inch out of it to look even better. And sometimes it's hard to figure out if something can be done in reality, or if it's just their perception of themselves. They may not be satisfied, or they may be terribly dissatisfied if you don't explain to them what it takes to look a certain way. For instance, you can tell them you can do a face lift, but they may not be thinking about the marks that can be left. And marks do show in some circumstances. And like a tummy tuck. Sure, you can get rid of a big tire around your middle, but you'll also have a scar. They have to realize what the trade-off is.

"Sometimes, it's hard to live up to your own idea of what perfection is. I'm very disappointed if my results aren't extremely good. And though it's not true in reality, I always wonder if I could have done more, even if it's not possible. But I'm learning to accept what the reality of the field is. You can only do so much.

"And as with any specialty, you're always afraid of a lawsuit, with the litigious climate that exists today. Even good results could end you up in court."

How Ernest DiGeronimo Got Started

"I grew up in a professional family, my father was a dentist, my mother was a nurse. Going from high school to college I never even questioned whether or not I should go into medicine. It was only *where* I should go.

"Originally, I was going to be a dentist. I figured I'd walk right into my father's practice and have it made. I went to Assumption College in Worcester, Massachusetts and graduated in 1970 with a B.S. in biology. At that time I was torn between medicine and dentistry. But 1970 was right in the middle of the Vietnam war and it became even more competitive to get into any dental or medical school. Being in school was one way of avoiding the draft.

"I did get into a dental school, but decided I really wanted to pursue medicine. And I knew I wanted to be a surgeon because, luckily, I was gifted with artistic talent in my hands. It was natural for me. While I was applying for dental school, I also sent out a few applications to foreign medical schools, in Spain, Italy, and Mexico. I ended up getting accepted at the University of Guadalajara in Mexico. I had a friend who was already there and he said it was great. So I decided to go.

"I finished in 1974. But because it was a foreign school, to get an equivalency rating with American schools at that time, you had to do what was called an externship, the "fifth pathway." I did the externship at Muhlenberg Hospital in Plainfield, New Jersey. That was one year.

"After I finished that, I was the equivalent of an M.D. in the United States. During that year I applied for residency programs. I was accepted into a program in Jersey City with the New Jersey

College of Medicine and Dentistry. I did two years of general surgery there. I had considered heart surgery, I figured they were the kings of the hill. Then I switched to being a neurosurgeon for a while. But after seeing all the people turning into vegetables and dying, I realized I wanted something a little less traumatic and severe. One of my jobs in general surgery was to notify the family of their loss and it was very draining.

"I met another doctor who had chosen plastic surgery and he highly recommended it. Your patients are healthy, not sick. You can choose the kind of surgery to do and schedule it when you want. There are very few emergencies in plastic surgery.

"My third year I switched to Englewood Hospital in New Jersey and then I applied to plastic surgery programs. I ended up at the University of Miami and worked with Dr. Ralph Millard, who is world famous. I did two years of plastic surgery there and after that I was a plastic surgeon. That was 1980.

"Right after that, I started in an office with another doctor, sharing office space for a little while. Now I have my own practice and rent out space to other doctors."

Expert Advice

"You need to be a people person, so people can feel comfortable talking to you. You also have to know how to handle emotions. For example, patients can be apprehensive about the healing process, which does take some time. And often you have family members to deal with, who might not think their relative should be having the procedure. And you have to know how to turn down a patient, if you don't think there'll be a significant benefit.

"Unless you're a natural at it, you shouldn't go into plastic surgery. It takes a while to build up a practice starting out. You have to do a good job for that good job to send you another patient. And you have to love it with a passion or you won't succeed at it."

●   ●   ●

FOR MORE INFORMATION

For a list of medical schools and general information on training, financial aid, and medicine as a career contact:

The American Medical Association (AMA)
515 N. State Street
Chicago, IL 60610

Association of American Medical Colleges
Section for Student Services
2450 N. Street, NW
Washington, DC 20037-1131

For information on osteopathic medicine as a career contact:

American Osteopathic Association
Department of Public Relations
142 East Ontario Street
Chicago, IL 60611

American Association of Colleges of Osteopathic Medicine
6110 Executive Blvd., Suite 405
Rockville, MD 20852

CHAPTER 2 Physician Assistants

📖 EDUCATION
A.A./A.S. Required
B.A./B.S. Recommended

$$$ SALARY/EARNINGS
$50,000 to $75,000

OVERVIEW

The physician assistant field is a fairly new one, starting just over 25 years ago. When the medics in the army came back from active duty with so much medical training and experience, there developed a strong need to utilize those valuable skills. Thus, the PA field was born.

As their job title implies, physician assistants support physicians, but at a much more advanced level than medical assistants (described in Chapter 5).

PAs are formally trained to perform many of the routine but time-consuming duties that usually fall to the physician. They take medical histories, examine patients, make preliminary diagnoses, treat minor injuries, and sometimes assist in surgery. In 35 states and the District of Columbia, PAs are allowed to prescribe medication.

Physician assistants always work under the supervision of a doctor, but the amount of supervision will vary depending upon the job setting. For instance, in a rural or inner-city clinic that is visited only once or twice a week by a physician, the PA will bear most of the responsibility, checking in with the doctor via telephone.

Some PAs will make house calls or visit patients in the hospital, then report back to the attending physician. PAs can also specialize–in orthopedics or pediatric care, for example.

JOB SETTINGS

Most PAs work in doctor's offices and clinics. Others work in hospitals. The rest work for public health clinics, nursing homes, prisons, and rehabilitation centers.

About one-third of all PAs provide health care to communities where physicians may be in limited supply.

TRAINING

Almost all states require physician assistants to complete a formal training program. Admission requirements to these programs vary, but most require at least two years of college and some work experience in the health care field. Most PAs will graduate with a bachelor's degree, some go on for a master's. A small few might receive an associate's degree or certificate.

The PA program itself generally lasts two years and can be found in four-year colleges and universities, medical schools, and schools of allied health. A few programs are offered at two-year community colleges and in hospitals.

SALARIES

Salaries vary by specialty, setting, geographic location, and years of experience. A survey conducted by the American Academy of Physician Assistants in 1993 showed that the average yearly salary for all PAs was between $50,000 and $55,000.

RELATED FIELDS

Other professions that provide direct patient care at the same level of skill as PAs include nurse practitioners, physical and occupation therapists, speech-language pathologists, and audiologists.

INTERVIEW

Sherry Crespo
Physician Assistant

Sherry Crespo has worked in a number of settings: departments of surgery in various hospitals, private practice for a surgeon, and most recently in the emergency room of a small community hospital.

What the Job's Really Like

"Your duties will depend on where you're working and for whom, and what you'll be asked to do will depend on the scope of the setting or the doctor's practice. Basically, a PA takes a history and examines the patient. Sometimes you have to do a complete exam, and sometimes, if you're working in an emergency room, for example, you might do a more focused exam relating only to their complaint. We could order tests–x-rays or blood tests–depending on what we think might be wrong with them. We wait until the results come back, then discuss them with the physician and see if there's anything else the physician wants to do or order. If the patient has something we need to treat, we can treat it to a certain extent. For example, if the patient has a fracture, we might splint it or cast it. If they have an abscess we would drain it. If they need surgery and you're working in the hospital, you might assist the surgeon in the operating room. But we are not the scrub nurses who are handing instruments to the surgeon; we have our hands in it, actually assisting with the procedure.

"PAs are not allowed to practice on our own, which is essentially the only thing we're not allowed to do. Anything else that the physician we work with allows us to do, we are allowed to do. We aren't always directly supervised, some things we can do on our own, but you always have to work under the auspices of a physician. You have to be able to discuss cases with physicians, even if it's only by phone. They have to at some point cosign the chart.

"This job at the ER has been a lot of fun. You see a lot of different problems patients come in with. You get exposure to different conditions and learn something new every day. The ER where I work is not a big trauma center and there's not that much of a diverse population. You won't get the big car accidents with people's hands sliced off or see a lot of head trauma, for instance. Those cases would be sent to a different hospital.

"You're up and down all day. You see a patient and sit down while you're writing up the chart, or you're on the phone between patients, calling the lab for results or x-ray or talking to physicians.

"I've worked all different shifts, from 11:00 P.M. to 7:00 A.M., from midnight to 8:00 A.M., from 4:00 P.M. to midnight. In this job I work 40 hours a week from noon to eight. And I cover weekends, too.

"If you're female, though, this job is a little bit tougher, because people tend to think you're a nurse. Patients, other nurses, and the physicians ask you to do things that are not really for you to do. In general, you don't get that level of recognition in this field that you would if you were male. If a male and female walk into a patient's room, the patient almost always automatically thinks that the male is the doctor, the female, the nurse. It's a stereotype. Even if I've already told a patient I'm the physician assistant, I might come into his room when he's on the phone with his family and hear him say he has to hang up now because the nurse just walked in.

"And there seems to be more of a camaraderie between the male physicians and the male PAs. They're taken under the physicians wing more, and more male PAs are encouraged to go on to medical school. Only female physicians have ever encouraged me to go on.

"And I think there's not a lot of recognition, in general, of the PA field. Even only six months after I graduated, I found I was not really that thrilled with the PA profession. Maybe it was the first job I had in surgery at a hospital. They had residents there and I think that whenever you have residents on the scene, you get stuck doing a lot of the junk work that nobody else wants to do. So if an IV needed to be started or blood needed to be drawn or they needed another assistant in the operating room, you'd be assigned to it. You get treated like the resident's assistant. I'm currently looking for another job and though there are jobs available in surgery, you know you're going to get stuck holding a retractor for another intern. Even though you've seen and done the procedure yourself a thousand times. I'd rather be doing the surgery myself or first assisting. Not second assisting alongside somebody who knows nothing. I've been out of school 13 years and they probably got out just this past June.

"It's better if you work for a physician in private practice. Then, I was his first assistant and we did all of the cases together. In a hospital, you can hope to find someone who will take a shine to you and take you under his or her wing. But it doesn't happen too often, because they're really there to teach the residents, not you.

"There's a lot of competition, too, between PAs and nurse practitioners. We vie for the same jobs and they have a lot more leeway and are able to set up their own private practices. PAs can't."

How Sherry Crespo Got Started

"I had gone to college, to NYU, and was about 20 when I graduated in 1978 with my B.A. When the diploma came I wondered what I was going to do with it. I had majored in biology and then you could teach or go into research. That was about it. I spent the next two years doing odd jobs, teaching high school equivalency, working in a butcher shop for a while, working in a bakery for a while. But my friends kept encouraging me to do something with my degree. One was in podiatry school, another dental school, but I knew I didn't want to look at people's feet or down their mouths for the rest of my life. Then I met someone at the bakery who was a PA. And I said, 'What's a PA?' This was 1979 and I'd never heard of it before.

"She told me what it was all about and it sounded like a good idea. The training was only two years and it didn't sound as if a lot of time and money had to be invested. You wouldn't have to give up your whole life the way you would with medicine.

"I went to Touro College in New York and got another bachelor's; this was a B.S. as a PA in 1982."

Expert Advice

"First of all, make sure you really want to be a PA and not an M.D. Know how strong your commitment is to medicine. The best thing to do would be to volunteer at a hospital, not as a candy striper, but working with a physician or a nurse or a PA you might know, so you can follow them around and learn what it is they really do. Or go to a private practice and volunteer in the office.

"I had been a candy striper for six months, and learned through that that I didn't want to be a nurse. And figure out how much patient care and the kind of patient care you really want to do. Nurses handle certain aspects of patient care, doctors and PAs handle different aspects.

"In nursing there are a lot of other roads. If you ever tire of patient care you can go into administration or teaching. But if you're a PA, you're stuck on a PA track. So make sure you know exactly what the different fields entail."

●   ●   ●

FOR MORE INFORMATION

A free brochure, *Physician Assistants, PArtners in Medicine*, is available from:

> American Academy of Physician Assistants
> 950 North Washington St.
> Alexandria, VA 22314

For a list of accredited programs and a catalog of individual PA training programs, contact:

> Association of Physician Assistant Programs
> 950 North Washington St.
> Alexandria, VA 22314

For eligibility requirements and a description of the Physician Assistant National Certifying Examination, write to:

> National Commission on Certification of Physician Assistants, Inc.
> 2845 Henderson Mill Rd., NE
> Atlanta, GA 30341

3 Registered Nurses

EDUCATION
B.A./B.S. Recommended
Other

$$$ SALARY/EARNINGS
$30,000 to $40,000

OVERVIEW

A wide range of career opportunities is open to registered nurses. Just as many medical doctors specialize, so do nurses. They can work with extremely ill people or with a well population. However, the two fields, medicine and nursing, though related, are very different, and it's easy to make a mistake when it comes time to choose.

If you like the scientific aspect–running chemical and laboratory tests, or doing dissections, for example—then medicine is the career you should choose. But if you prefer hands-on contact with patients, or like concerning yourself with healthy foods, exercise, doing all the right things to stay healthy, and you like to teach, then nursing should be your career.

There are a lot of nurses who became nurses because they didn't think they could get into medical school–but they don't end up enjoying nursing. Their interest really was in the scientific aspect, not the social aspect. And, there are physicians out there (even though they'd probably never admit it) who really hate science and would have preferred to become nurses. Make sure you understand what's involved before you choose.

JOB SETTINGS

Approximately 68 percent of all nurses work in hospital settings. Others work in clinics, private doctors' offices, nursing homes, training rooms, first aid stations at sporting events, summer camps, school infirmaries, rehabilitation centers, outpatient centers, and even prisons. They work in rural areas, such as on Indian reservations, in Alaska, or in the Appalachian Mountains, or around the world on cruise ships, with the Armed Forces, the Foreign Service, the Peace Corps, or the Red Cross. Some also, in much the same way a doctor does, set up their own office and work in private practice. Others even make home visits.

Nurses who become teachers instruct future nurses in hospital training programs, in two-year community colleges, in four-year colleges and universities, and in master's and doctorate programs. They can also work in technical schools in programs that prepare licensed practical nurses or in a large hospital, welcoming newly employed nurses with orientation and training to hospital procedures.

EDUCATION
B.A./B.S. Required
Post Graduate Recommended

$$$ SALARY/EARNINGS
$40,000 to $75,000+

Nursing Specialties

Below is a list of all the different areas in which a nurse can choose to specialize:

FAMILY NURSING, working with every age range from neonatal and pediatrics to geriatrics. In addition to their license to be a registered nurse, these professionals go on to become nurse practitioners or nurse midwives.

HOSPITAL NURSING encompasses a whole range of specialties.

The Emergency Room (ER): Here patients come in from the street, on their own, or brought in by the police or paramedics. They can be suffering from a variety of traumas: anything from a broken bone, gunshot wound, or serious burn to a heart attack or a stroke.

Intensive Care Unit (ICU)/Cardiac Care Unit (CCU): Here patients are in critical condition and require more intensive, one-on-one care.

Medical/Surgical: Here patients are suffering from a variety of illnesses and ailments or are recovering from surgery.

Obstetrics and Gynecology (OB/GYN): Here you'll find the maternity ward, where women deliver their babies, and the nursery, for newborn infants. Women also are admitted to this part of the hospital for surgery or other procedures.

The Operating Room (OR): Here surgeons, OR nurses, nurse anesthetists, and other professional staff work as a team during operations.

Out-Patient Departments/Clinics: Here patients are seen who are not sick enough to be admitted to the hospital. They might need a follow-up visit to check their medication, or physical therapy, or a session with a counselor. After their appointment they return home.

Psychiatric Ward: Here patients are suffering from a variety of emotional problems or illnesses, such as depression or schizophrenia.

ADMINISTRATION, directing the activities of a department, hospital, or other setting. There is less hands-on patient care at this level; nursing administrators deal with hiring and firing, budgets, schedules, and a score of other issues.

NURSE EDUCATORS train other nurses or provide information and instruction to patients and staff on a variety of subjects.

COUNSELING NURSES work with a basically well population, providing support and information.

TRAINING

At present, there are four different ways you can become a registered nurse, or R.N.:

1. Through a two-year community college, earning an associate's degree in nursing;

2. Through a three-year hospital-based nursing school, earning a diploma;

3. Through a four-year university program, resulting in the Bachelor's of Science degree in nursing, or the B.S.N., as it is commonly called;

4. And, for those who already have a bachelor's degree in a different subject, there is a "generic" master's degree in nursing, a two- to three-year program beyond the bachelor's degree.

These days, and certainly in the future, the B.S.N. is being considered the minimum qualification for a satisfying career. The two-year associate's degree and the three-year hospital-based diploma programs are very quickly closing down throughout the country and student nurses are being encouraged to enroll in four-year universities.

For many nursing specialties, it is essential to also earn a master's degree or an advanced certificate; and for some nurses, those who wish to teach, for example, a Ph.D., or doctorate, in nursing is required.

After schooling, new graduates are expected to take a licensing exam, for the basic R.N. and for any of the various specialty areas.

WORKING CONDITIONS

Working conditions for nurses vary tremendously, depending upon the setting in which they choose to work. A nurse's schedule in a hospital setting is probably one of the most difficult. Although they generally work 40 hours a week, hospital nurses are expected to rotate shifts, and their hours could fall in the middle of the night, on the weekends, or on holidays.

Administrators, educators, and nurses who work in outpatient departments or clinics usually put in more normal hours.

Duties also vary according to the setting. For example, an ER nurse will deal with any kind of medical crisis; a sports medicine nurse will see only injuries common to athletes or other active patients.

Hospital nurses spend a great deal of their time on their feet, walking miles of hospital corridors, bending, and lifting. A nurse in the Foreign Service will travel around the world, working in an embassy infirmary with diplomats and their families.

JOB OUTLOOK

In general, employment opportunities for nurses are excellent. Specifically, a number of fields are experiencing extreme shortages, and there the chances for employment are much better than average. Here are a few examples:

In the past, most nurses earned their R.N. through a three-year hospital-based training program. But these programs are being slowly phased out and more and more nurses go directly into a four-year university to earn their B.S.N. This means that there will be more and more openings at the university level for nurse educators. Universities are already having difficulty recruiting enough teachers because of the low pay nursing educators generally receive. If you decide you would like to teach, and you've completed your higher degrees and have practiced in the field for several years, chances are you'll be able to find a job at the institution of your choice.

Because of health reform, health administration is opening up for nurses beyond the acute-care hospital. There will be a lot of different facilities–a variety of clinics, hospices, family planning centers, HMOs–where nursing administrators will find satisfying employment.

The job outlook for nurse midwives and nurse practitioners is excellent. With all the health care reform being planned, eventually physicians won't make as much money performing normal, routine duties. Their skills will be left to surgery and other complicated procedures and the skills of midwives and practitioners will be utilized more. In essence, costs will be kept down and everyone will save money.

But cost is not the only factor ensuring a good job outlook. There are many regions in the country that don't attract enough physicians. There are also some patient populations, such as the elderly or inner-city teens, that are being neglected. Midwives and practitioners are in even more demand to fill in in these areas.

SALARIES

Salaries will vary depending upon the organization you're employed with; they could range from only a small allowance in the Peace Corps to a more substantial income with the Foreign Service, for example.

With a few exceptions—nurse anesthetists, for example—hospital floor nurses are among the lowest paid of all nursing professionals. And some would argue that it's very unfair, because floor nurses also work the hardest of all the nursing careers.

Salaries do increase depending upon your level of education and the years of experience you have accumulated.

Because there is a great demand for nurse midwives and nurse practitioners, salaries are very high, if not the highest in the nursing profession. In fact, a midwife or practitioner can go into private practice and make about the same salary a doctor with a general practice would. This can run to six figures but, of course, depends on the area of the country in which you live and how much competition there is.

Traditionally, educators have always been the lowest paid professionals. First-year nurses graduating with a B.S.N. will generally earn more than their professors do. A nurse can make a lot more money outside an educational setting. Those who do decide to follow a career in nursing education are obviously not doing it for the money.

In addition to a high degree of job satisfaction, most administrators find the financial compensation to be more than fair. Depending upon the setting and your rank, your salary could range from $30,000 to $125,000 a year.

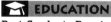

EDUCATION
Post Graduate Required

$$$ SALARY/EARNINGS
$40,000 to $75,000+

NURSE PRACTITIONERS

The nurse practitioner profession was designed more than 30 years ago to provide health care to people who didn't have access to physicians. And in some settings today (in rural villages, for example), nurse practitioners are still the only providers. They are legally licensed to prescribe medication in most states, and fully trained to fill in for pediatricians, obstetricians, and general practice physicians. In urban areas, practitioners work with physicians, providing a comprehensive health care package.

Practitioners focus their attention on a patient's common problems, freeing up time for the physician who is trained more to correct serious ailments. Nurse practitioners are not as disease-oriented; they try to prevent diseases, and if a disease is not readily correctable, they teach patients how to live with it. Nurse practitioners find work in city hospitals, clinics, and private doctors' offices; in rural areas, such as on Indian reservations, in

Alaska, or in the Appalachian Mountains; or around the world with the armed forces or the Foreign Service.

They can also, in much the same way a doctor does, set up their own office and work in private practice. Some nurse midwives and nurse practitioners even make home visits.

Training for Nurse Practitioners

Nurse practitioners study in special programs above the R.N. or B.S.N., receiving master's degrees and additional training. They also take special licensing exams for their specialties.

RELATED FIELDS

Workers in other occupations with responsibilities and duties similar to those of registered nurses are physician assistants, LPNs, physical and occupational therapists, and paramedics.

INTERVIEW

Bobbie Campbell
Sports Medicine Nurse

Sports medicine nurses often work as part of a team, with physicians and surgeons and physical therapists. They attend to both professional and amateur athletes, from Olympic ice skaters and professional ballet dancers, to the neighborhood soccer or Little League team.

Bobbie Campbell works in a private sports medicine clinic that is owned by a physician and a physical therapist. She has been a sports nurse for close to 25 years.

What the Job's Really Like

"Sports medicine is a sub-specialty of orthopedic medicine and deals primarily with injuries received during athletic activities. Sports medicine nurses care for patients suffering from strains, sprains, torn ligaments and muscles, fractures, and dislocations.

"It's the job of the sports medicine nurse to take a patient's history, assist the doctor with his or her treatment plan, and to educate the patient so future injuries can be avoided.

"I work about 36 hours a week. My hours can vary but they're usually Monday through Friday. I can arrive at 7 A.M. to a full schedule of patients. I'll escort them to the exam room, take a history, and do a brief screening. If necessary, I'll take their blood pressure and interview them about how they got their injury. I work with the doctor and when he goes to examine a patient I go with him. I write down everything he says and take notes for the patient. After the doctor leaves the room, I go over everything the doctor told the patient–the diagnosis, the plan for treatment, what they're supposed to do at home. I might give him samples of medication and explain the side effects–there's a lot of explanation to the patient. If needed I might also give an injection or take an x-ray.

"You have a lot of patient contact and generally you are dealing with a healthy and well-motivated population. I really like being able to share knowledge and educate people to prevent injuries.

"The hours are pleasurable too, much better than hospital work. The job is varied, there are a lot of different aspects to it. I work with different age groups and I get to incorporate a lot of the general knowledge I learned in my nursing program. You can take your education and skills and use them often. And you get to go to the ballet and sporting events.

"The only pressure I can think of is that most of the patients are in a hurry to get well. They're anxious to get back to their sport, and they want to get back *now*! That can be a great incentive, but it can also be a pressure. Bodies can heal only so quickly."

How Bobbie Campbell Got Started

"I always loved sports when I was a kid, but I wasn't a great athlete. Later, when I decided to become a nurse and I learned about the sport medicine specialty in my nursing program, I realized it would be a great way to combine my two interests. I started working in a hospital. One of the doctors there and a physical therapist decided to open their own clinic and I was thrilled when they asked me to join their staff."

Expert Advice

"First, you should be interested in a healthy lifestyle. And you have to want to work with patients; you're not going to be behind a desk. You have to be able to talk to patients and explain and teach. It's a teamwork approach. You work with the doctor and the physical therapist.

"You should also be able to do more than one thing at once–it's demanding. You might be working with the patient and then there's a telephone call, and at the same time the doctor is asking you to do something and you have to take an x-ray. It can all pile up at once and you have to have communication skills and the ability to delegate.

"Then, make sure you get involved with sports. If you can't participate for some reason, then get involved in athletic training. Get down to the training room and work with the coaches. Learn what the athletes need. Volunteer your time at local sporting events. Be a team manager. This is how you find out if it's for you. I've known kids who really got involved, then went on to become athletic trainers, physical therapists, nurses, and doctors. Take basic anatomy and physiology courses to see if it appeals to you. And definitely get a B.S.N. I would even suggest going on afterward for an advanced nurse practitioner degree. More doors will be open to you. The three-year hospital-based R.N. programs are fewer and fewer."

INTERVIEW

Stephie Morin
Certified Nurse Midwife

Stephie Morin has been a certified nurse midwife (R.N., C.N.M.) since 1986.

What the Job's Really Like

"A nurse midwife is trained in all areas of normal obstetrics, well-woman gynecological care, care of the newborn, and care of normal healthy women throughout their childbearing cycle, and afterward, too. In the United States, most midwives work in hospitals, but some work in birthing centers and some do home care.

"I work with a group of other midwives; our midwifery service is employed by the hospital and we also work with a group of physicians. Occasionally I travel to various community-based health centers but all the births I attend are in the hospital.

"A woman comes in for prenatal care at the health center. She'll see me for her first visit, which I hope will be early on in her pregnancy. I'll take a health history and I'll spend time getting to know her, giving her information about our service, about her pregnancy. I'll do some blood work, a physical exam, decide if any tests are needed, make any referrals, to a nutritionist, for example, or sometimes to a social worker, then I'll set up her next visit with me.

"During follow-up appointments we talk about how she's feeling, if the baby's moving yet–and we always listen to the baby's heart and measure the belly to see how it's growing.

"When my patient goes into labor, either I or one of my coworkers will meet her at the hospital. We'll evaluate her baby and her labor with different monitoring devices. We support her through the different stages of labor—a nurse will be there, too, and a doctor is always available in case of complications. And if the woman wants any medication, we're able to give it to her.

"After the baby is born, we have follow-up visits to teach her about newborn care and what to expect from her body as she recovers from the delivery.

"Delivering a baby can be a difficult time and the women appreciate the help you give them. You get really close to your patients; some come back for their second babies and you become almost a part of their family. I've even had quite a few women name their babies after me. They send pictures and you get to see how your namesake grows up. It's a real honor.

"But people have their babies all times of the day and night and on weekends. You have to be prepared to work in the middle of the night, you lose sleep sometimes and you put in long hours. But the rewards more than make up for it."

How Stephie Morin Got Started

"When I was just out of high school I met a nurse who was going to become a nurse midwife and that was the first I had heard of the career. At the same time, a woman I knew was going to have a baby and I got to be at the birth. It just clicked and I knew that's what I wanted to do.

"There are different way to become a midwife. My university program combined an R.N. with midwifery training and a master's degree in nursing. If you're not a nurse when you start the program it takes three years.

"But you don't have to be a nurse to be a midwife. Non-nurse midwives are called lay midwives, or empirical midwives, depending upon the region. There are restrictions in different states, and non-certified nurse midwives may not be licensed to the same degree or even recognized–it depends on the state."

Expert Advice

"You have to be a people person with a deep respect and understanding of the birthing process. You also have to be able to work as part of a team."

INTERVIEW

Bertha Lovelace
Nurse Anesthetist

Bertha Lovelace is the chief nurse anesthetist at a Cleveland, Ohio-based world-famous referral center for all sorts of medical illnesses. She has been a nurse for close to 30 years.

What the Job's Really Like

"Basically, a nurse anesthetist is responsible for keeping the patient anesthetized and free of pain during an operation. She or he is also responsible for bringing the patient back to a state of wakefulness afterward. Generally, we use sodium pentothal or other medications that are called inhalation agents, or breathing agents.

"Before a patient's surgery we meet with him, in a pre-operative clearance, to ask about his physical well-being, any history of surgery or encounters with anesthetics and if he has any allergies, or when he ate last.

"During the surgery we monitor the patient's vital signs and adjust the anesthetic according to the patient response.

"Because I am the chief nurse anesthetist I am also a clinical instructor of student nurses.

"We work as part of a team, designing a plan for the patient with the anesthesiologist (M.D.). The anesthesiologists act as the directors of the operating rooms and, in addition to the OR nurse and the surgeon, there is a nurse anesthetist with the patient at all times.

"I really get a sense of success after each operation, knowing I kept the patient pain-free and then was able to awaken him in a timely fashion afterward. There's a great sense of contributing a major part to the patient's comfort level.

"Also, you are working with a team of decision-making people. You have to be able to make split-second decisions; there's not a lot of leeway. It's stimulating. And because we're a teaching hospital we're always learning something new.

"I also like that it's one-on-one patient care. You deal with one case at a time. This career also offers a challenge that regular floor nursing didn't offer me.

"There is also a very nice financial reward. Salaries for nurse anesthetists are generally 40 to 50 percent higher than for floor nurses.

"The pressures are entwined with the pleasures. Every patient responds differently so you must always be on your toes, thinking about your next step—if you need to give more anesthesia, for example.

"There's also pressure when you work with very sick patients. Then your anesthesia has to be customized."

How Bertha Lovelace Got Started

"After the four-year B.S.N. program I went into an accredited nurse anesthetist program in a school of nurse anesthesia. This program took two and a half years to complete. In addition, I had to have one year critical care experience before I could enter the anesthetist program. Most nurses graduate and work one year before going for nurse anesthetist training. So, altogether, you would have seven and a half years training and experience before you could be a nurse anesthetist."

Expert Advice

"There are certain qualities you should have. I'll list them for you. You have to be:

Organized

Cost-conscious

A quick thinker

Even-tempered

Sensitive to the needs of others

An effective communicator, both verbally and in writing

And committed to your work."

INTERVIEW

Brad Potts
Nurse Practitioner

Brad experimented with a lot of different careers–oceanography, respiratory therapy, even auto mechanics–before he discovered nursing.

What the Job's Really Like

"A nurse practitioner evaluates a patient's total health care needs. My patients are anywhere from two weeks old to elderly. Initially, we do a head-to-toe physical and a complete health assessment. If a patient comes in with a specific complaint that's complicated and would require complicated intervention, we can refer him or her to a physician, or if it's a common health problem, we can handle it ourselves.

"There are always too many people to see and not enough time to spend with them, so you can feel pulled from all directions. It's a universal problem. So many people need health care and there are just not enough people and not enough time to take care of everyone the way you'd like.

"And the paperwork is terrible. You have to document everything. You worry about medical/legal issues. You don't want to end up in court. I have malpractice insurance through my job, but I also carry an additional policy for more protection.

These days, everyone seems to be lawsuit-happy and anyone who had any contact, even if they just said 'hello,' could be named in the lawsuit. It's gotten out of hand."

How Brad Potts Got Started

"I have a B.S.N. and a M.S. in primary care. I chose a family practice because I really like being able to take care of the whole family–the newborns, Mom and Dad, Grandmom and Granddad, and aunts and uncles and sisters and brothers–because health care is more than just the individual. Where you come from, the culture you're in, the beliefs of your parents or grandparents–it's all a big influence. If one person is sick, it affects everybody. When I know what's going on in the family, it helps me deal with all the family members. If a baby is sick, for example, and I'm seeing Grandmother, I know she might be very upset about the baby and might not be sleeping well."

Expert Advice

"Being a nurse, who also happens to be a man, can cause some awkward moments," Brad says. "An obstacle that I'm always trying to overcome is that I'm not a *male nurse*, I'm a nurse practitioner and I see all patients, men and women.

"If you're a male thinking about becoming a nurse practitioner, you have to be prepared to stand your ground. In nursing school I was always assigned to male patients. I used to have to ask to get a female patient assignment. My being there was awkward for my instructors, who were all women; they didn't know how to deal with it.

"And, sometimes, because I'm a male, patients assume I must be a doctor. I'm always correcting that impression–I think it's important that people understand the difference between doctors and nurses. But I'm more likely to run into discrimination by my colleagues–female nurses–than by my patients.

"I've had to go out to the people who schedule the appointments and instruct them not to steer female patients to female providers and male patients to the males. I talk to my colleagues on a regular basis about this.

"The advantage I do see to being a man who is a nurse is that I can be a role model for young men. Oftentimes, a male might think that nursing would be something he'd like to do, but because it's not what men *usually do*, he might shy away. At least they can see me out there, a typical man, who's doing nursing as his chosen career."

FOR MORE INFORMATION

The National League for Nursing publishes a variety of nursing and nursing education materials, including a list of nursing schools and information on financial aid. For a complete list of NLN publications, write to them for a career information brochure.

National League for Nursing (NLN)
Communications Department
350 Hudson Street
New York, NY 10014

For a list of B.S.N. and graduate programs, write to:

American Association for Colleges of Nursing
1 Dupont Circle, Suite 503
Washington, DC 20036

Information on career opportunities as a registered nurse is available from:

American Nurses Association
600 Maryland Ave. SW, Suite 100 West
Washington, DC 20024-2571

Most professional associations have prepared pamphlets and information packets including up-to-date salary figures, education requirements, and job outlooks. Write to any of the following specialty organizations for their material.

Advocates for Child Psychiatric Nursing
437 Twin Bay Drive
Pensacola, FL 32534

American College of Nurse Midwives
1522 K Street, NW, Suite 1000
Washington, DC 20005

American College of Sports Medicine (ACSM)
Member and Chapter Services Department
P.O. Box 1440
Indianapolis, IN 46206

American Health Care Association
1201 L St. NW
Washington, DC 20005-4014

The American Organization of Nurse Executives
840 North Lakeshore Drive
Chicago, IL 60611

American Psychological Association
750 First Street, NE
Washington, DC 20002-4242

Association for the Care of Children's Health
7910 Woodmont Ave., Suite 300
Bethesda, MD 20814

Association of Community Health Nursing Educators
c/o 64 Neron Place
New Orleans, LA 70118

Association of Women's Health, Obstetric, and Neonatal Nurses
409 12th Street, SW, Suite 300
Washington, DC 20024

Council on Graduate Education for Administration in Nursing
Duquesne University
630 College Hall
Pittsburgh, PA 15282

Department of Veterans Affairs
Title 38 Employment Division
810 Vermont Ave., NW
Washington, DC 20420

National Alliance of Nurse Practitioners
325 Pennsylvania Avenue, SE
Washington, DC 20003-1100

National Association of Orthopedic Nurses (NAON)
Box 56
East Holly Avenue
Pitman, NJ 08071

National Nursing Staff Development Organization
437 Twin Bay Drive
Pensacola, Florida 32534

Orthopedic Certification Board (ONCB)
Box 56
East Holly Avenue
Pitman, NJ 08071

Society for Education and Research in Psychiatric-Mental
  Health Nursing
437 Twin Bay Drive
Pensacola, FL 32534

CHAPTER 4

Emergency Medical Technicians and Paramedics

OVERVIEW

Emergency medical technicians, or EMTs as they are commonly called, and paramedics provide emergency medical services to victims of accidents and disasters and to anyone suffering from a medical crisis or trauma.

EMTs and paramedics work for private ambulance companies, in emergency rooms in some hospitals, and for city or county agencies. But fire departments are, by far, the largest employer of emergency medical service workers. This is because more and more fire departments across the country have combined firefighting with rescue services. Each fire department has to make sure a large number, if not all, of its firefighters are also trained emergency medical technicians and paramedics. When the 911 call comes in and the tones start sounding throughout the station, these professionals must be able to respond to any kind of emergency, whether a fire, a car accident, or a medical crisis. Firefighting as a career is covered in depth in *On the Job: Real People Working in Service Businesses*.

EDUCATION
H. S. Required
Other

$$$ SALARY/EARNINGS
Minimum wage to $40,000

The Role of the Emergency Medical Technician

EMTs are versed in the basics of first aid and life-saving. They learn CPR, patient handling, extrication of victims–from wrecked cars to earthquake sites–the basics of medical illnesses and medical injuries.

Essentially, EMTs provide basic life-support. They are expected to arrive on the scene and take care of a patient until the paramedics get there. If the EMTs and paramedics arrive together, then the EMT would assist the paramedic.

If the EMT is working in an area of the country where higher level paramedics are not a part of the team, he or she would then be responsible for getting the patient to the hospital.

An EMT might also be responsible for driving the ambulance.

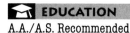

EDUCATION
A.A./A.S. Recommended

$$$ SALARY/EARNINGS
$12,000 to $50,000

The Role of the Paramedic

A paramedic has to be an EMT before becoming a paramedic. Paramedics are trained in very sophisticated, advanced levels of life-support. Their goal is to keep a patient alive and they function in the field as an extension to a physician. They are the pre-hospital hands, eyes, and ears of the doctor and have to be able to assess a situation and react the way a doctor would.

When possible, paramedics contact the hospital and let the doctor know what they have done for the patient. Some ambulances or rescue trucks have the capability of transmitting medical data such as EKGs by radio to the hospital. At this point, the doctor could let the paramedics know if there is anything else that should be done before bringing in the patient.

Paramedics have a strong relationship with physicians, who have learned over time to trust the paramedics' training and expertise.

The Duties and Limitations

Although EMTs perform very valuable services to patients in the field, statistics have shown that the more advanced the forms of treatment, the better the patient's chances of survival are. This is why paramedical training beyond the EMT level was begun.

For example, if someone has a cardiac arrest at home, the EMT can go to the house, start CPR, put him on a stretcher, give him oxygen, and hope the patient pulls through. With only a four to six minute grace period before the brain becomes permanently damaged from lack of oxygen, the actions of the EMT help, but in many cases are not enough.

The paramedic can function in the field the way the doctor would in the emergency room. Paramedics can defibrillate, oxygenate, and administer some drugs right on the spot. The less time the patient is down, the less time he spends not breathing, the higher his chances of recovery. Paramedics strive to deliver fast and effective intervention.

Another important role of EMTs and paramedics is to restore order and calm people down. Many calls they go on do not really require their level of care, but they do require their emotional or psychological support. The EMT and paramedic are there to help the patient through whatever he needs, even if all that involves is some hand holding and a smile.

In general, EMTs and paramedics don't really have to know *what's* wrong with someone, but they do have to be able to recognize when something *is* wrong. Emergency medical personnel do not carry cat scans, MRIs, and x-ray machines with them; they can't diagnose. But they can have a good feel for what's happening and be smart enough to identify when something needs further attention.

The Excitement and the Stress

EMTs and paramedics employed by a fire department will work shifts just as the firefighters do. The most common is 24 hours on with 48 hours off.

When not out on a call, the emergency medical worker will spend time at the fire station with his or her coworkers. But the time is not spent relaxing; it's spent waiting. As experts will tell you, you don't schedule the work, the work schedules you. You'll always be waiting for the alarms to go off. You might have to interrupt a meal, your sleep, your shower, getting dressed, going to the bathroom.

When you hear the tones, you run for the truck or ambulance and you get in as quickly as possible. If you're driving, you have to know where you're going and, if you don't know the area well, you have to be able to read maps. There's a lot of pressure to get to the scene fast. In this kind of occupation lives can be lost if you waste time.

There'll be lights flashing and a lot of noise with the sirens going off, and some find that exciting and fun. The air is electrified and invigorating and it's nice to see traffic get out of your way, but it is also dangerous. Just because 40 cars pull over doesn't mean that the 41st will. You can easily get into an accident yourself.

Every call will be different. It could be a grisly train wreck, or a false alarm. You'll have bad days with 20 calls or a day with just five. You never know.

When you get to the scene, you'll see people waving, you'll see police, crowds, and one of the stressors is realizing they're all waiting for you. When you get out of the truck, all the eyes are on you. You can't afford to look frightened or uncertain. You're expected to have a good idea what's wrong and to do the right thing.

You work hard and quickly to stabilize the patient and when you have, you get him or her into the hospital. On the way you call ahead and let them know to expect you. At the hospital you usually stay a little while, dealing with relatives and hospital personnel.

You never know who your patient is going to be. You might have to deal with drunks or hostile people or situations that are potentially violent. Sometimes you think you're going on a call for someone who is sick, but when you get there it turns out to be something else–maybe someone who is acting crazy, waving a gun around. Sometimes there are police to help you, sometimes they're busy and they can't. Every now and then an EMT or paramedic is killed in the line of duty.

There is also the danger of contracting a contagious disease from a patient.

The rewards come from helping people and saving lives. But it's not just the major incidents that are satisfying. Sometimes it's the small things, helping someone who's down and out and feels that no one care about him. And sometimes people are scared and making them feel better makes you feel better.

TRAINING

EMTs can generally be trained in 6 to 12 weeks, through a community college. During the course of their program, they spend time observing in hospitals and gaining practical experience riding with an ambulance crew.

To become certified, EMTs are given a practical exam through the school and a written exam through the state.

Once you have become a certified EMT, you can then go on to paramedic school. Most programs are offered through community colleges and that is the most popular route to go, though there are a few private paramedic training schools here and there. The training for a paramedic could take anywhere from two to three semesters or two years, depending upon the state in which you live.

The course of study for a paramedic is a full curriculum with coursework including anatomy, physiology, pharmacology, the administration and interpretation of electrocardiograms (EKGs), medical diagnoses, handling cardiac arrests, defibrillation, and all the related medical subjects.

Paramedic trainees spend a lot of time in hospitals learning advanced techniques. They work in operating rooms with anesthesiologists learning intubation, the process of inserting a tube into a patient's windpipe. They also spend time on hospital critical care floors, learning from the nurses how to take care of patients. Trainees also participate in birthings and learn about pediatrics.

EMTs and paramedics working as firefighters must learn about the different lifesaving equipment available to them, including extrication devices, air splints, pediatric immobilizers, suction units, and portable defibrillating and EKG machines.

In addition, to keep their certification current, emergency medical service workers also must participate in continuing education classes, often offered by their employers.

SALARIES

Depending upon the region of the country, EMTs working for a private ambulance company in a small town can make as low as $5 to $10 an hour. In the dual role of firefighter and EMT, they can make anywhere from $25,000 to $38,000 a year, again depending upon the area of the country. Those figures can rise substantially over the years as experience increases.

Paramedics working independently of a fire department could make anywhere from $12,000 to $20,000 a year. Combined paramedic/firefighters generally start in the mid to high 20s, or even in the 30s or low 40s in some high-cost cities, and can go as high as $50,000 or more per year.

RELATED FIELDS

Other workers in occupations that require quick and level-headed reactions to life-or-death situations are police officers, firefighters, air traffic controllers, workers in other health occupations, and members of the Armed Forces.

INTERVIEW

Tania Maxwell
Emergency Medical Technician

Becoming a firefighter had been Tania's childhood dream, a dream she was able to see come true in 1987. She has been an EMT since 1989 and plans to study to become a paramedic.

What the Job's Really Like

"EMTs help the paramedics out, making their job easier. We do basic life-saving, CPR when necessary, apply bandages, get the medications for the paramedics to administer–all the basics.

"We get a chance to see a lot of things, we get a chance to be in on everything because the EMTs go wherever the paramedics go. We get a chance to work with the people, up close and personal.

"We're involved with everything that has to do with saving lives. Calls we could go out on could be heart attacks, people feeling faint, people having babies, shootings, stabbings, slip and falls, or car accidents. We sometimes even get called out for minor things, a cut finger or a scratched knee.

"But what I enjoy most is being around the people. After the paramedics have done their work and taken the patient to the hospital, as an EMT I get to stay around and talk to the family, explain what we're doing and reassure them that we have some of the best paramedics in the state, in the nation. We're going to do everything we can to make sure that patient gets better. They couldn't be in better hands.

"But it's frustrating when there's nothing you can do. Where I live we have a lot of swimming pools, and therefore drownings. The worst part is rolling up on a little kid who was left unattended and has fallen into the pool. You do everything you possibly can, but sometimes it's still not enough.

"But I try to think about the flip side, that it's always joyful to bring a life into this world when we deliver a new baby and that we save a lot more lives than we lose.

"As a woman EMT/firefighter, I don't want anyone to have to pull my weight. Now I think that because I've been doing this job for more than seven years, I've already proven myself. I am able to do my job and do it effectively, but at the beginning, I felt as if I had to work harder.

"The guys didn't make me feel that way, it was all me. They're like my big brothers. They look out for you and make sure nothing happens to you. Everything is on the buddy system. You know that your big brother is right there with you."

How Tania Maxwell Got Started

Tania's neighbor was the chief of her hometown fire department. "As a kid I used to see his truck in the neighborhood, in front of his house and it fascinated me. He talked to me about the profession, inspired and encouraged me.

"When I graduated high school I went to the community college and took an EMT course, then applied to the fire department. But getting the job wasn't the end of my training, it was just the beginning."

Expert Advice

"To be the very best at whatever you choose to do, whether it's firefighter, EMT, or paramedic, and to remember that hard work and perseverance make everything go well. This advice can go for anyone, really, it's universal. If the mind can perceive it, you can achieve it. If you think big enough, you can do anything."

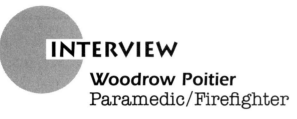

INTERVIEW

Woodrow Poitier
Paramedic/Firefighter

Woodrow Poitier became a paramedic first before becoming a fire-fighter. In fact, he was in the first group of 12–affectionately called the Dirty Dozen–his city hired when the program was started back in 1975.

What the Job's Really Like

"My main duty is to preserve life and limb. Whenever we're called for an emergency we go out and try to take care of the problem. Every call is different.

"I also function as a paramedic supervisor. The paramedic supervisor only goes on certain calls, normally those that involve trauma or calls involving children. That's not to bust anybody's chops, but just to make sure the job is done properly.

"In addition to the emergency calls, there are the reports we have to write and we also have to stock the truck and make sure the equipment is always ready to go. Everyday there's an assignment to take care of.

"We also have controlled drugs on the trucks such as Valium and morphine and we have to be very careful about that.

"I've delivered about a total of 14 babies, most of them in the back of ambulances on the interstate. One lady named her child after me.

"I've worked shootings, stabbings, cuttings, drownings, you name it. You get the drunk drivers who cause so many accidents, but most of the time they don't even get hurt. The Lord takes care of children, fools, and drunks. Children are resilient. Even if they get hurt, they seem to have the ability to jump right back.

"I've seen calls where everything has gone right, we have dynamite paramedics on the scene, yet you can't save the victim. Then other times, everything seems to go wrong, you can't get an IV started, nothing seems to be working, and yet he lives.

"There's no rhyme or reason. I do know the paramedics do a good job. Even if you are able to help only one person in a 24 hour period, it makes it worth it.

"It's satisfying work. I really do enjoy being a paramedic. After all these years I'm still gung ho. Even when I'm off duty and I'm at home and hear the sirens go by, it gets the adrenalin going.

"I like most being able to help people. Every emergency is different and, believe it or not, you come into people's homes, their lives, and the positive energy you input always seems to have a positive result, and that's really, really rewarding.

"Then there are times when you're down, if a child has died for example, but you take the good with the bad.

"We go out on a lot of calls and most of them are legitimate calls, but a lot of them are not. These are calls we don't deem as emergency calls. Like the guy who's had a toothache for three days and he decides to call you at three o'clock in the morning because he can't fall asleep and he wants you to do something. Or the guy who stubbed his toe. Some people feel that if they call us and go to the hospital on a stretcher they'll get treated more quickly in the emergency room. There's a lot of misuse of the system. But when you get the legitimate calls it makes it all worthwhile."

How Woodrow Poitier Got Started

"My family owns a funeral home and when I was a kid, we also ran an ambulance service. That's how I got my first exposure to the profession. I acted as an EMT, doing first aid and that sort of thing before there were any official training programs available. When our family went out of the ambulance business, I went to work for a private ambulance company. At the time, the para-medical field was spanking brand new, just coming into play. The ambulance company said they'd give me and all my drivers a job if we went to EMT school. So I did, then on to paramedic school, both at a local community college. I worked for the ambulance company from 1971 to 1975, then joined the fire department as a paramedic. After I was hired, they sent me for firefighting training.

"The pay was one thing that attracted me, but the other was being able to help people, trying to make some kind of differ-ence. I wanted to let people who were hurt know there was someone out there who cared."

Expert Advice

"If they want a rewarding job and one that actually helps people, than this is the job to go into. But you have to stay in school and get that piece of paper.

"And of course it would help to have some sort of desire to go into the medical field. If they don't want to go to great lengths to become a doctor, the paramedic field would be the way to do it."

INTERVIEW

Harry Small
Commander of Emergency Medical Services

Commander Harry Small oversees 3 supervisors and 65 paramedics at a large city fire department.

What the Job's Really Like

"I used to be out there as a paramedic, but my job now is to make sure that all the EMTs and paramedics have everything they need to do their job. My duties cover several different areas. I make sure the EMTs and paramedics are properly trained. I arrange for their classes and I do some of the continuing education training myself.

"I oversee the warehouse operation, ordering supplies and buying equipment. I have to make sure the trucks are properly stocked.

"I plan a budget and administer it. I keep records on all personnel and equipment and the maintenance of vehicles. I deal with conflicts, between staff and hospitals for example, and listen to the problems of my employees. Whatever is wrong, I try to fix it. I also deal with anyone in the general public who calls us with a problem.

"There are a lot of meetings to attend and state guidelines to follow. Because paramedics can come into contact with contagious diseases, we have excessive amounts of documentation to handle if someone has been exposed–procedures for testing, compliance with state regulations, that sort of thing.

"And paramedics have to write reports for each call they go on. The supervisors have to make sure they are filed properly and I have to review all of this paperwork.

"Mainly, my job is to support that system that's out there working and make sure that system can continue to work.

"I really miss working in the field. This job is five days a week, 40 hours, a very standard job, not as exciting. You don't get the chance to do all the things you could do before. Periodically, I go out and ride with the team just to have a part in it, but it's not the same. I have to get my satisfaction from watching them do well. If they do well then I can feel good. You have to learn to enjoy your success through other people–that's a manager's role."

How Harry Small Got Started

"I started in 1976 as a volunteer firefighter. I worked my way through the ranks as a firefighter/paramedic and became Commander in 1991."

Expert Advice

"Education is crucial these days. They should think about earning a college degree–in EMS and fire science–because that's becoming more and more important. There aren't many bachelor degree programs now, it's mainly at the associate's level, but in coming years there will be more and more four-year programs. And for administration, it's also a good idea to have a business background, take a B.A. or even a master's in business management.

"In fire departments where there is an EMS division they should also make sure they have an EMS background. New leaders will start coming from the paramedic corps—this was rare in the past.

"And when opportunities present themselves to learn new skills, through your organization or on your own, take advantage of it. You'll want to study management, human development, handling conflict, anything related to your work. If it's not made available, seek your own. You need to grow and to learn more than your job because the best paramedic or firefighter won't necessarily make the best administrator or manager. The technician doesn't automatically become an administrator."

• • •

FOR MORE INFORMATION

General information about EMTs and paramedics is available from:

> National Association of Emergency Medical Technicians
> 9140 Ward Parkway
> Kansas City, MO 64114

Information concerning training courses, registration, and job opportunities can be obtained by writing to the State Emergency Medical Service Director, listed in your phone book.

The Red Cross offers courses in basic first aid and CPR. You can find an office near you by looking in your phone book. The address for their national headquarters is:

> American Red Cross
> National Headquarters
> 17th & D Streets, NW
> Washington, DC 20006

High schools often offer a health occupations program that will allow students to get a taste of all the different medical paths.

Students in this program take medical skills classes in the tenth grade. In the eleventh or twelfth grade they spend 36 weeks studying medical courses, going on field trips to hospitals and community centers, and riding with ambulances or fire/rescue trucks. By the time they finish, they will know if being a paramedic or a doctor or an emergency room nurse would be the career they'd prefer.

This program is open to all students dedicated to pursuing a career in health occupations. Students in this program must also be members of HOSA–Health Occupations Students of America.

For more information contact the high school guidance counselor or health occupations teacher or write to:

> Health Occupations Students of America (HOSA)
> 6309 N. O'Connor Rd., Suite 215 LB117
> Irving, TX 75039-3510

5

Medical Technicians

OVERVIEW

The term "medical technician" has a broad scope, covering several different job titles and a wide range of responsibilities. The *OOH* lists the following technician job titles within the field of medicine:

Medical Assistant

Medical Laboratory Technologist/Technician

Medical Records Technician

Medical Secretary

Each occupation is distinctly different, carrying job-specific duties, training requirements, working conditions, and salaries.

EDUCATION

H.S. Required
On-the-Job Training Possible
A.A./A.S. Recommended

$$$ SALARY/EARNINGS

$12,000 to $20,000

Medical Assistants

The duties of a medical assistant will vary from setting to setting. Those working in a small doctor's office might perform a variety of tasks, clerical as well as technical. In a larger office with a number of employees, the medical assistant's duties could be more specialized. The interview included in this chapter will give you a good idea of what a jack-of-all-trades medical support position entails.

TRAINING FOR MEDICAL ASSISTANTS. Positions are available to medical assistants who have had no formal training, although there are more opportunities and better paying positions for those who have gone through some sort of training program. Training is available through vocational programs as well as community colleges and four-year colleges and universities. Programs can take from one to two years and result in a diploma, certificate, or associate's degree.

Two agencies recognized by the U.S. Department of Education accredit programs in medical assisting: The American Medical Association's Committee on Allied Health Education and Accreditation (CAHEA) and the Accrediting Bureau of Health Education School (ABHES).

Information on the different programs can be obtained from the addresses listed at the end of this chapter and by speaking directly to the school or program you are considering attending.

EDUCATION
B.A./B.S. Required
Post Graduate Recommended

$$$ SALARY/EARNINGS
$20,000 to $30,000

EDUCATION
H.S. Required
On-the-Job Training Possible
A.A./A.S. Recommended

$$$ SALARY/EARNINGS
$20,000 to $30,000

Medical Laboratory Technologists and Technicians

Laboratory testing plays an important role in the diagnosis and treatment of disease. Medical laboratory technicians and technologists, also called clinical laboratory technicians and technologists, perform these tests.

These professionals analyze body fluids, tissues, and cells. Utilizing a range of equipment, they look for parasites, bacteria, or other microorganisms.

TRAINING FOR MEDICAL LABORATORY TECHNOLO-GISTS/TECHNICIANS. Medical technologists usually have at least a bachelor's degree in medical technology or one of the life sciences. Some have a combination of formal education and work experience. Universities and hospitals offer these training programs.

A master's degree is necessary for research, teaching, administration, and for certain specialties within medical technology.

Medical laboratory technicians usually have an associate's degree from a community college or a diploma or certificate from a vocational education training program. A few technicians learn on the job.

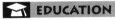

EDUCATION
A.A./A.S. Recommended

$$$ SALARY/EARNINGS
$20,000 to $30,000

Medical Records Technicians

Every contact a medical professional has with a patient is recorded into the patient's chart. The job of the medical records technician is to assemble the chart, make sure it is complete and that all forms are identified and signed. Sometimes, they verify diagnoses when necessary with the physician, or talk to other staff to update the file.

Medical records technicians use a coding system for each diagnosis and procedure. This helps with billing and insurance claims. All patient information is input into computer files.

Medical records technicians usually work in hospitals and clinics, though sometimes they are employed in large private practices. They usually work a 40 hour week, from Monday through Friday.

TRAINING FOR MEDICAL RECORDS TECHNICIANS.

Most medical records technicians usually enter the field with two years of training through a program awarding an associate's degree. These programs are offered at community colleges and include course work in medical terminology, legal aspects of medical records, anatomy, physiology, statistics, databases, quality assurance methods, and computer training.

The American Health Information Management Association (AHIMA) also offers an independent study program. (The address for more information on this program is listed at the end of this chapter.)

Most employers prefer to hire Accredited Record Technicians. Accreditation is obtained by passing a written exam offered by AHIMA, but to take the examination, you must be a graduate of a program accredited by the Committee on Allied Health Education and Accreditation (CAHEA) of the American Medical Association, or a graduate of the independent study program AHIMA offers.

EDUCATION
H.S. Required
A.A./A.S. Recommended

$$$ SALARY/EARNINGS
$20,000 to $30,000

Medical Secretaries

Secretaries are responsible for coordinating office activities and keeping administrative operations under control. Specific duties vary according to job setting. Medical secretaries working in a private doctor's office or in a particular hospital department or floor could be responsible for patient charts, correspondence, filing, scheduling, and a variety of other administrative duties.

Secretaries held more than 3 million jobs in 1992. Of that number, 234,000 are medical secretaries.

TRAINING FOR MEDICAL SECRETARIES. High school graduates may qualify for entry-level secretarial positions, provided they possess basic office skills including word processing and other computer skills. Formal training will lead to higher paying positions. Training is available through high school courses, vocational education programs, and community colleges, as well as on-the-job training.

SALARIES FOR MEDICAL TECHNICIANS

Salaries for all sectors of the medical technician field vary widely, depending upon geographic location, job setting, the education of the worker, and the number of years experience. The following figures are averages compiled from a variety of surveys conducted by various professional associations. For more detailed information refer to the *OOH*.

MEDICAL ASSISTANT. With 2 years experience or less the average salary is $13,715. With 11 years of experience or more, salaries average $20,885.

MEDICAL LABORATORY TECHNOLOGIST/TECHNICIAN. Average annual earnings runs about $26,000. Half of those surveyed earned between $19,000 and $32,000. The lowest 10 percent earned less than $14,664 and the top 10 percent earned more than $39,000.

MEDICAL RECORDS TECHNICIAN. Accredited record technicians who work as coders earn on the average $11.30 an hour. Unaccredited coders average $9.77 an hour. Supervisors average $29,599 a year. Medical records technicians working for the federal government in nonsupervisory and supervisory positions averaged $22,008 in 1993.

MEDICAL SECRETARY: The average annual salary for all secretaries, regardless of specialty, was $26,700 in 1992.

RELATED FIELDS

Workers in other medical support occupations include hospital admitting clerks, pharmacy technicians, dental assistants, and physical and occupational therapy aides.

Workers who perform duties similar to those performed by medical laboratory technicians and technologists include chemists, science technicians, crime laboratory analysts, food testers, and veterinary laboratory technicians.

Occupations related to medical secretary work include bookkeepers, receptionists, clerks, legal secretaries, and human resource officers.

Occupations utilizing skills similar to those needed by medical record technicians include medical secretaries, medical transcribers, medical writers, and medical illustrators.

INTERVIEW
Deanna Fusco
Medical Secretary/Office Manager

Deanna Fusco works in a private practice with Dr. Steven Magilin, a general surgeon in Miami, Florida. She started in 1989 as a medical secretary and is now in charge of every aspect within the doctor's office.

What's the Job Really Like?

"My duties within this office include almost everything, with the exception of doing the insurance billing and the actual surgery. I make the appointments, I verify the patients' insurance and make sure they have all the proper paperwork. I make the doctor's daily schedule, letting him know what meetings he has to go to, which patients he'll be seeing, which procedures he'll be doing. Because he's a surgeon, he has to take emergency room call at several hospitals and I'm in charge of making sure that's always covered if he's not available. I do his weekly schedule, and I schedule all his surgery and other procedures, both in the hospital and in the office. Basically, I let him know where he has to be every moment of every day, as long as he's in my charge, then I send him home to his wife.

"I also type consult letters for the doctor. When a doctor refers a patient to us, as a courtesy, I send him a consult letter, letting him know the doctor saw the patient and what his diagnosis and treatment plan is.

"I answer a lot of patient questions over the telephone. Mostly, it's putting someone at ease before a surgical procedure or diagnostic testing. And I let them know how to prepare themselves before the procedure, eating lightly, for example.

"I am the first contact that the patients have, either by telephone or by walking into the office. I also take the patient into the examination room and help prepare him for his exam. And I also assist the doctor in the examination rooms, helping him with dressing changes, handing him instruments, and making sure he has the equipment he needs. Normally, a medical secretary wouldn't do that, but it's a small office, only the doctor and myself, and that's why my job encompasses so many different things.

"Because it's a surgical practice, it's a more transient set of patients. Someone will come with an appendix, for example. The doctor will take out the appendix, follow that patient post-operatively, but once that patient is released from care, nine times out of ten, he wouldn't need to come back, unless he has another problem that's within the doctor's field.

"I also take care of the operative reports, which is the doctor's dictation after a surgical procedure. We get reports on pathology and it's my job to make sure the doctor sees them and that they then get incorporated into the patient's chart. Filing is another one of my duties. I'm in charge of all the patients' files. I pull the charts for patients the doctor will see on any particular day and make sure that everything is in the chart that's supposed to be there.

"I make sure the office complies with OSHA requirements and I also make sure that we comply with the state's biomedical waste regulations.

"I order office supplies and all the supplies the doctor needs and I keep an inventory of the supplies. I even take care of the magazines in the reception area, making sure they're current and in order.

"In the mornings, the doctor is always in the hospital doing procedures or surgery, so I'm able to do all the paper work and filing then.

"My day doesn't start getting really hectic until he comes in about one o'clock. For the last part of the day, when we have patients in the office, some days I would label it the craziest thing in the world. I'm running from room to room, answering telephones, making sure the patients have what they need, making sure the doctor has what he needs, and sometimes, I'm ready to pull my hair out of my head.

"But I wouldn't have it any other way, though. I love it. And I love having the patient contact; I'm a people person. Maybe it's rewarding to me, too, because I know I can do it. It takes a special kind of person to be able to walk in here and do all of the different things. You have to be extremely flexible and you have to be what I call 'slightly left of center.' The doctor is a perfectionist and he expects that out of me. And I have come to expect no less than that from myself.

"The only downside to the job is that you never know when an emergency is going to walk in, or another physician is going to call you up and say 'I have somebody in my office and I need to send him over immediately.' It might happen at the end of the day when I'm on my way out the door to go to a movie, but you stay late when you have to. Even though I work, basically, nine to five, I can't always count on getting out of the office at five. And though I'm not expected to work on a weekend, sometimes I come in on a Sunday if I need to catch up with my paperwork."

How Deanna Fusco Got Started

"For 10 or 12 years I worked in customer service and I did very well because I'm a people person. I worked in several different retail settings. Floor and tiling, appliance repair. But customer service is customer service, no matter where you're doing it. I do, however, prefer medical settings over retail ones. Probably because it's very technical. There's only so much you can learn about a piece of fabric or carpet or how to stop a toilet from running. But with the medical field, you're saving lives and constantly learning. Things are always changing and I like that change.

"I left the retail field and worked in a hospital's outpatient department as a registration clerk. The office manager who was here before me wanted to semi-retire and go to part-time. She used to speak with me over the phone, booking the appointments, so she recommended me to interview with the doctor, to see if we could get along and if I would like to work in a doctor's office. And that's how I got to be here.

"I started out as just a secretary, but as other employees shifted jobs, moved away and left, my duties increased. The doctor saw that I was intelligent and that I could learn and that I had the ability to deal with the people, so he decided that, as long as I was happy, he'd let me take on more and more responsibility. All my training was on-the-job. The doctor taught me everything I know. It's been wonderful. As a boss, he's the best, as a surgeon he's very competent, he cares for his patients and if I ever had to have any surgery, I'd want him to do it.

"The move from the hospital to the doctor's office was a step up in pay as well. I had been earning about $16,000 a year and my salary went to $18,500 with the new job. Currently, I earn $23,800 a year."

Expert Advice

"Know what you want to do. If you're interested in the medical aspects and want to be a medical assistant, for example, then go to school and get the diploma or certificate. It would be very difficult to find a doctor who would take someone off the street who knew nothing, and then teach him. Plus, when you have the education, it ensures that you'll get a higher salary."

●　　●　　●

FOR MORE INFORMATION

Information about career opportunities, CAHEA-accredited education programs in medical assisting, and the Certified Medical Assistant Exam is available from:

The American Association of Medical Assistants
20 North Wacker Dr., Suite 1575
Chicago, Il 60606-2903

Information about career opportunities and the Registered Medical Assistant certification exam is available from:

Registered Medical Assistants of American Medical Technologists
710 Higgins Rd.
Park Ridge, IL 60068-5765

For a list of ABHES-accredited educational programs in medical assisting, contact:

Accrediting Bureau of Health Education Schools
Oak Manor Office
29089 U.S. 20 West
Elkhart, IN 46514

For information on career opportunities and certification for clinical/medical laboratory technicians, contact:

American Society for Medical Technology
7910 Woodmont Ave., Suite 1301
Bethesda, MD 20814

American Society of Clinical Pathologists
Board of Registry
P.O. Box 12277
Chicago, IL 60612

International Society for Clinical Laboratory Technology
818 Olive St., Suite 918
St. Louis, MO 63101

National Certification Agency for Medical Laboratory Personnel
7910 Woodmont Ave., Suite 1301
Bethesda, MD 20814

For a list of educational programs accredited by CAHEA for clinical laboratory personnel, contact:

Committee on Allied Health Education and Accreditation
515 North State St.
Chicago, IL 60610

For a list of training programs for medical laboratory technicians accredited by ABHES, contact:

Secretary–ABHES
29089 U.S. 20
West Elkhart, IN 46514

Information about employment opportunities in Department of Veterans Affairs medical centers is available from local medical centers and also:

Title 38 Employment Division (054D)
Department of Veterans Affairs
810 Vermont Ave., NW
Washington, DC 20420

For information on secretarial careers, contact:

Professional Secretaries International
10502 N.W. Ambassador Dr.
Kansas City, MO 64195-0404

For information on careers in medical record technology, contact:

American Health Information Management Association
919 N. Michigan Ave., Suite 1400
Chicago, IL 60611

A list of CAHEA-accredited programs is available from:

American Medical Association
Division of Allied Health Education and Accreditation
515 N. State St.
Chicago, IL 60610

CHAPTER 6 Dental Technicians

OVERVIEW

Just as with the medical technician careers investigated in the previous chapter, the term "dental technician" refers to a range of trained professionals who are right hand helpers to the dentist or oral surgeon.

In addition to the career of dentist (explored in Chapter 10), the *OOH* lists the following technician job titles within the field of dentistry:

Dental Assistant

Dental Ceramist/Dental Laboratory Technician

Dental Hygienist

Each occupation is distinctly different, carrying job-specific duties, training requirements, working conditions, and salaries.

⬛ EDUCATION
H. S. Required
On the Job Training Possible
AA/AS Recommended

$$$ SALARY/EARNINGS
$12,000 to $20,000

Dental Assistants

Dental assistants can be assigned to one of three areas of responsibility, although many offices require that the assistant be skilled in all three.

1. *At chairside*, working closely with the dentist and patient. In this area, dental assistants perform the following duties:

Make patients as comfortable as possible

Prepare patients for treatment

Obtain dental records

Hand instruments and other materials to the dentist

Keep patients' mouths dry using suction or other devices

Sterilize and disinfect instruments and equipment

Prepare tray setups for dental procedures

Provide postoperative instruction

Provide instruction in oral health care to patients

Some dental assistants assigned to chairside duties might also perform these additional functions:

Prepare materials for making impressions and restorations

Expose radiographs

Process dental x-ray film

Remove sutures

Apply anesthetic and/or preventative sealants to patients' gums and teeth

2. In the office laboratory, dental assistants:

Make casts of the teeth or mouth from impressions taken by the dentists

Clean and polish removable appliances

Make temporary crowns

This area of responsibility differs from the full laboratory duties of a dental laboratory technician or dental ceramist. See the job description for laboratory technicians below.

3. *Front office dental assistants* take care of a range of clerical duties such as:

Make appointments

Receive patients

Keep treatment records

Send bills and process payments

Order dental supplies and materials

TRAINING FOR DENTAL ASSISTANTS. Most assistants are trained on-the-job, though many graduate from dental assisting programs offered by community colleges, trade schools, and technical institutes.

Training programs include classroom, laboratory, and pre-clinical instruction in dental assisting skills and related theory. Students also gain practical experience in dental schools, clinics, or dental offices.

Most programs take one year or less to complete and lead to a certificate or diploma. Two-year programs through community colleges offer an associate's degree. Certification is available through the Dental Assisting National Board (the address is listed at the end of this chapter), but is not required for employment.

EDUCATION

H.S. Required
On-the-Job Training Possible
A.A./A.S. Recommended

$$$ SALARY/EARNINGS

Minimum wage to $30,000

Dental Laboratory Technicians/Dental Ceramists

Dental laboratory technicians are like pharmacists; they fill prescriptions. But their prescriptions come from dentists and are for crowns, bridges, dentures, and other dental devices.

They work with plaster, wax, and porcelain, using small handheld tools through a variety of the stages required to produce the device. In some laboratories, dental laboratory technicians perform all stages of the work; in other labs the different stages are assigned to different technicians.

Technicians also may specialize in one of five areas: orthodontic appliances, crown and bridge, complete dentures, partial dentures, or ceramics.

Technicians who make porcelain and acrylic restorations are called dental ceramists.

TRAINING FOR DENTAL LABORATORY TECHNICIANS. Most dental laboratory technicians learn their craft on the job. However, formal training programs are available through community colleges, vocational-technical institutes, and the Armed Forces.

The training process to reach complete proficiency can take an average of three to four years, depending upon the individual's aptitude and ambition. However, it may take a few more years to be recognized as an accomplished technician.

EDUCATION
A.A./A.S. Required
B.A./B.S. Recommended

$$$ SALARY/EARNINGS
$30,000 to $40,000

Dental Hygienists

Dental hygienists examine patients' teeth and gums, record abnormalities, remove calculus, stain, and plaque, take and develop x-rays, place temporary fillings and periodontal dressings, remove sutures, and, in some states, administer local anesthetics and nitrous oxide.

Dental hygienists also instruct patients in good oral hygiene. Some develop and promote community dental health programs.

Dental hygienists use hand and rotary instruments to clean teeth, x-ray machines, syringes, and models of teeth.

TRAINING FOR DENTAL HYGIENISTS.   A dental hygienist must be licensed by the state in which he or she chooses to practice. To receive a license, a hygienist first must graduate from an accredited school and pass both a written and a clinical exam.

Most programs lead to an associate's degree, though some offer a bachelor's. A small few lead to a master's degree. The associate's degree is sufficient for practice in a dental office. A higher degree is usually required for research, teaching, or clinical practice in public or school health programs.

JOB OUTLOOK FOR DENTAL TECHNICIANS

Jobs for dental assistants and dental hygienists are expected to grow at a fast rate in response to increasing demand for dental care.

Job prospects for dental laboratory technicians, while still good, are not expected to be as plentiful as for the previously mentioned job titles. The main reason for this is that with increased dental hygiene awareness, it is estimated there will be less need for dental appliances. Basically, people are keeping their teeth longer.

SALARIES FOR DENTAL TECHNICIANS

DENTAL ASSISTANT.   According to the American Dental Association, dental assistants who work 32 hours a week or more average over $330 a week. Average hourly earnings run about $9.20.

DENTAL CERAMIST/DENTAL LABORATORY TECHNICIAN. Data is limited, but in 1991 average hourly earnings were reported at $13.30. Trainees can start out at only a little better than minimum wage.

DENTAL HYGIENIST. Salaries for dental hygienists are often double that of the dental assistant. According to a survey conducted by the American Dental Association, earnings averaged about $609 a week in 1991 (the latest available data). Hourly rates averaged about $18.90.

Salaries for dental hygienists vary greatly depending upon the geographic location and other factors such as education and experience. A dental hygienist can be paid hourly, by the day, or by the patient, as well as a yearly salary. Successful hygienists with a few years experience under their belts can earn up to $200 or $250 a day.

RELATED FIELDS

Fields related to dental assisting include medical assistants, physical and occupational therapy assistants, pharmacy assistants/technicians, and veterinary assistants/technicians.

Fields where work is performed similar to that of dental laboratory technicians include arch-support technicians, orthotics technicians (braces and surgical supports), prosthetics technicians (artificial limbs and appliances), opticians, and ophthalmic laboratory technicians.

Occupations related to that of the dental hygienist, a field involved in supporting a doctor in his or her responsibilities, include physician assistant, nurse practitioner, and other medical, ophthalmic, and dental assistants.

INTERVIEW
Eileen Edgecomb
Dental Hygienist

Eileen Edgecomb works with two other hygienists in a private group practice owned by three dentists. She has been in that office since 1990.

What the Job's Really Like

"Hygienists take any necessary x-rays, update medical histories, if the patient has been in the office before, or take a history if it's a new patient.

"You are not only just cleaning their teeth, you are finding out if there are any areas of special concern to point out to the doctor when he comes in for his examination. You're checking the gums to see if there are any signs of gum disease, you're instructing the patient on home care, brushing, flossing, and so on.

"And one other thing I've found over the years is that sometimes you are, in a way, a friend to the patient. Sometimes they just need someone to talk to, to reassure them that the appointment is not going to be as terrible as they're thinking it will be. Sometimes you have to just be an ear.

"It's very important in my field of medicine to have compassion. So many times people are afraid of the dentist, and whereas I have never had a bad dental experience, I understand that there are people who have. They have very real fears and I can try to sympathize. Many times I've done more listening than cleaning. You need to be a people person, you need to be able to talk to people and to be compassionate.

"And you can't take it personally when they attack you. They told us in hygiene school we'd better be able to handle a lot of negative emotion. I've been called names, I've been given dirty looks and told I must like to inflict pain. Sometimes the hardest part of the job is the person, not the mouth.

"But sometimes, the nicest part of the job is also the person. You get that 'thank you', people who really appreciate what you're doing. And when you see that person sitting in the chair with his teeth shining and he leaves happy, you get your reward right there.

"There are some downsides to watch out for, though. If you don't sit correctly, you can get neck and back trouble. You can also develop, if you have the criteria, carpal tunnel syndrome. You can also get, like what I've developed, tendinitis.

"Another downside can be the doctor you're working for. If you don't have a doctor who is compassionate, and really cares about the quality of his work, but is only out to make all the money he can and has that godlike attitude, it can be really hard. I've worked in offices where I've only lasted a couple of months because of that.

"What's kept me going is that I enjoy the people, and that I'm single and self-supporting. I'm very grateful that I had some sort of foresight years ago to pick a respectable and well-paid profession.

"Hygiene, as well as dentistry, has a high burnout rate. There are not going to be a lot, like me, at it for over 20 years, because of all the negatives.

"But for me the positives have outweighed the negatives. There are the patients, the doctor, when he's nice, the salary. And when you've helped someone. Say he has a broken tooth and you fix it, or he has a lot of staining and you polish his teeth. Afterwards, your patients feel so much better about themselves. If they have brighter smiles and can chew their food better and have healthier mouths, it feels good to be able to help that process.

"I know that I'm providing a good service for the public, even if they don't want to be there, they feel good when it's over. I try to make it easy for them. If I make it hard on them, they won't want to come back. I'm not one of those hygienists who criticizes and condemns. I ask people to try their best. I arm them with the information they need and the rest is up to them."

How Eileen Edgecomb Got Started

"My mother started taking my brother and me to her dentist when I was about four. I had very positive experiences there. I can still remember my two hygienists' names, even after all these years. My mother started working for our family dentist as a dental assistant when I was in the ninth grade and we became friends of the family. I babysat his kids, we went to his house for parties, and I just kind of fell into the office. I admired the hygienists and looked up to them.

"I had wanted a profession that didn't require a lot of education, that paid well, that had decent hours, that maybe I could work four days a week. And I thought also that if I got married and had children it would be something I could do part-time, because the salary is very good.

"I had also wanted to get into a profession where I could help people, but I was a little too emotional for medicine. One of the advantages of dentistry is that people don't die. After all, it's just your teeth.

"I went to a two-year community college in Edison, New Jersey, and got an associate's degree in applied sciences and graduated in June of 1975. The program was a combination of classroom and hands-on training. There was a clinic right in the school so I worked on patients there."

Expert Advice

"You have to be good at sciences and health-related sciences and it's also a good idea to take some psychology courses because you'll be dealing with people. And as I said before, it's very important to be a people person, to have compassion."

●   ●   ●

FOR MORE INFORMATION

Information about career opportunities, scholarships, accredited dental assistant programs, and requirements for certification is available from:

American Dental Assistants Association
203 N. LaSalle, Suite 1320
Chicago, IL 60601-1225

Commission on Dental Accreditation
American Dental Association
211 E. Chicago Ave., Suite 1814
Chicago, IL 60611

Dental Assisting National Board, Inc.
216 E. Ontario St.
Chicago, IL 60611

For information about training to become a dental laboratory technician and a list of approved schools contact:

Commission on Dental Accreditation
American Dental Association
211 E. Chicago Ave., Suite 1814
Chicago, IL 60611

For information on career opportunities in commercial laboratories and for requirements for certification, contact:

National Association of Dental Laboratories
3801 Mt. Vernon Ave.
Alexandria, VA 22305

For information on a career in dental hygiene and the educational requirements to enter this occupation, contact:

Division of Professional Development
American Dental Hygienists' Association
444 N Michigan Ave., Suite 3400
Chicago, IL 60611

7 Dietitians and Nutritionists

OVERVIEW

Historically, dietitians have been thought of as professionals who work in hospitals. Nutritionists have traditionally worked in the community on an out-patient basis, counseling for nutritional problems or weight loss. They also work in health food stores, helping customers with nutritional concerns. But basically, the two terms carry the same weight, as long as both professionals have gone through similar training programs and are licensed by the state.

Dietitians or nutritionists find employment in hospitals, schools, day care centers, summer camps, hotels, natural food stores, and weight-loss clinics. They can also set themselves up in private practice.

🎓 EDUCATION
B.A/B.S. Required
Post Graduate Recommended

💲💲💲 SALARY/EARNINGS
$20,000 to $40,000

The Role of Registered Dietitians and Nutritionists

There are several different kinds of dietitians with a wide variety of duties.

CLINICAL DIETITIANS generally work in a hospital setting in a patient-oriented role. Each dietitian is usually assigned one or two floors, about 50 patients per dietitian.

Clinical dietitians visit patients, review their medical records, and evaluate their nutritional status to determine what would be the best diet for them to be on depending on what their medical problems are. They would look at the chart to see what kind of lab results they had and what they were admitted for. They would interview the patients, asking about their diet history, what they usually eat, if they've been following any special diets, if they've lost weight recently, if they have any trouble swallowing, chewing, and so on.

That information is then recorded in the medical record before it gets processed in the diet office, where the menus are originated. Afterward, it is passed on to the kitchen so patients can be fed three times a day.

Dietitians work with regular diets or design diets with restrictions for patients with ailments such as diabetes, renal or cardiac problems, or cancer.

SPECIALIZED DIETITIANS work with special needs patients such as in kidney dialysis centers where diet plays a major role in the treatment of the patient. They deal with tube feedings or parenteral nutrition, when a patient is fed a concentrated formula of carbohydrates and protein through a large vein.

ADMINISTRATIVE DIETITIANS oversee the entire food service operation including purchasing, storing, and preparing food and other functions of the kitchen.

COMMUNITY DIETITIANS, or nutritionists as they are sometimes called, work with patients on an outpatient basis, in a health food store, clinic, or private practice. They counsel patients to help them lose weight or bring down their cholesterol level, deal with food allergies, or a variety of other concerns.

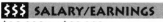 **EDUCATION**
A.A./A.S. Required
B.A./B.S. Recommended

$$$ SALARY/EARNINGS
$12,000 to $20,000

Dietetic Technicians

Registered dietitians, especially in large and busy hospitals, depend on the help of registered dietetic technicians, or diet techs, as they are called. Most diet techs are clinically oriented and do basic screenings of patients, review medical records, and document their findings in the chart. They generally handle the less complicated cases, leaving specialized patient needs to the registered dietitian.

Diet techs can also work in nursing homes, overseeing the food service operation or working in the kitchen.

Diet Aides/Nutrition Assistants

⬛ EDUCATION
H.S. Required
On-the-Job Training Possible

$$$ SALARY/EARNINGS
Minimum Wage to $12,000

Aides or assistants function in a clerical role. They write the patients' name and room number on the menus, pass them out to the patients on the floors, and wait while the different preferences are checked. They then review the menus, making sure they've been marked properly.

TRAINING FOR DIETITIANS

A dietitian must have a four-year degree in nutrition and foods from an accredited university.

Coursework will cover a lot of science–biology, chemistry, physiology–and nutrition, math, foods, and food science.

A six- to nine-month supervised internship is also required. Some programs allow the internship to run concurrently with the senior year; in other programs the internship can be started only after graduation.

After the internship you are eligible to take a registration exam put out by the American Dietetic Association, the national professional organization. After passing the exam, you are then a registered dietitian.

Some dietitians go on for a master's degree, especially if they are interested in more administrative positions or want to maintain their competitiveness for jobs.

Training for Diet Techs

Diet techs usually earn a two-year degree in foods and nutrition at a community college. They are then eligible to take an exam administered by the American Dietetic Association to become a registered dietetic technician. Many then find jobs and continue to study on the weekends to earn their four-year degree.

Training for Diet Aides

Diet aides and nutrition assistants usually have no formal training in foods and nutrition. They must have a high school diploma and have good written and verbal skills. The work is mainly clerical and most are trained on the job.

Becoming a diet aide is a good way to get a taste for the profession, so to speak. After spending some time in a hospital food department, you can then decide if you want to go on for further training.

THE HOURS

Your shifts will vary depending upon the setting, but for the most part dietitians avoid weekend work and the late night and overnight shifts that many nurses must deal with. But some dietitians are on-call over the weekend and must come in for emergencies.

Diet techs and assistants aren't as lucky and generally they do pull regular weekend duty.

For diet aides, the earliest shift would start about 5:30 in the morning in order to help get out breakfast. They would finish up about 2:30 in the afternoon. The latest shift would finish at about 7:30 in the evening after the dinner meal is over.

SALARIES

As with most professions, salaries vary depending upon the region of the country in which you work and the size of the hiring institution's budget. Registered dietitians usually are paid an annual salary. For entry-level candidates, that could fall into the mid 20s and go up with more experience.

Administrators, depending upon their responsibilities, could earn from $30,000 to $80,000 a year.

Diet techs generally start out in the low 20s. Diet aides are usually paid hourly, from $5.50 to $7 or so.

The benefits of working in a hospital usually make up for the low pay. This includes good health care plans, pensions, vacation days, sick leave, and holidays and personal days.

RELATED FIELDS

Dietitians and nutritionists apply the principles of nutrition in a variety of settings. Workers with duties similar to those of administrative dietitians include home economists and food service managers. Nurses and health educators often provide services related to those of community dietitians.

INTERVIEW

Emily Friedland
Dietitian

Emily Friedland is the assistant director of food and nutrition at a large private hospital. She has a B.S. in nutrition and foods from Cornell University and a M.A. in food service management from New York University. She has been working in the field for more than 20 years.

What the Job's Really Like

"I am responsible for the entire department; we have about 100 employees. Our department is made up of different sections—patient feeding, cafeteria feeding, visitor coffee shop, and clinical nutrition. In the clinical nutrition area I directly supervise a total of 25 dietitians, diet techs, and nutrition aides.

"I review their work, maintain and update a diet manual, which is all the different diets our patients might be on, and write and implement policies and procedures. My job is varied, it's different each day. We have an in-service training program, so every month there are one or two classes we present, and we are continually measuring the quality of our performance.

"I enjoy being in a management position. You never know what you're going to face when you walk in the door in the morning. There are always different crises that come up—a piece of equipment is broken, or someone didn't show up to work. In the food service industry you are committed to getting those three meals out every day and if someone doesn't show up you can't just say, 'well we're short-handed so we won't serve breakfast today.' You have to put out a product no matter what the inputs are.

"There's a lot of variety. There's always new cases, different needs, it doesn't get boring.

"I just wished we had more respect in the health care industry. But I think it's coming. The stereotype of the gray-haired lady in the school cafeteria is changing. People are recognizing that nutrition does have a great influence on health–treatment of disease and also prevention of disease.

"And the training is changing, too. It's more clinically oriented. Things that the dietitian was doing 18, 20 years ago when I first started are what the diet tech does now. The registered dietitian is getting more involved in the complicated cases now. As our dietitians are being more and more specialty trained and the physicians see that this person really know what he's talking about, there will be more and more respect.

"We're also lobbying very hard to have our services covered in the new health care reform. Right now nutrition services are not covered by insurance programs and sometimes people are reluctant to spend $60 or whatever to consult a dietitian. But on the other hand, they'll go into a health food store and spend hundreds of dollars on vitamins they don't need and that are only going to go right through their systems. They'll pay for that but they won't pay for a licensed practitioner to really put them straight as far as what they need to be doing.

"And I don't think for the amount of education and training we have that we are recognized and compensated as much as some of the other health care professionals.

"But the upside is it's a great job if you enjoy working in a health care setting, working with people, but don't want to do hands-on care. And if you enjoy the relationship between food and health, you're able to put that into practice."

How Emily Friedland Got Started

"In high school I always enjoyed home economics and I had a teacher who introduced me to the field. I didn't start out as a nutrition major, I was a little scared off by all the science requirements. But I did take a nutrition class my first semester at college and decided that I really liked it and quickly changed my major from consumer economics to foods and nutrition.

"I also worked in a nursing home in a kitchen as a food service worker during summers while in college."

Expert Advice

"I'd advise anyone wanting to pursue this career to go ahead and get the proper education and training. You can start out as a diet tech through a two-year program, to see if it's what you'd like, and then go on for your bachelor's degree."

● ● ●

FOR MORE INFORMATION

For a list of academic programs, scholarships, and other information about this field contact:

The American Dietetic Association
216 West Jackson Blvd.
Chicago, IL 60606-6995

CHAPTER 8 Physical and Occupational Therapists

OVERVIEW

Physical and occupational therapists help people with physical and emotional limitations to reach their full potential.

The purpose of physical therapy is to correct musculoskeletal dysfunction and problems with movement. The physical therapist works independently, evaluating patients, designing and implementing treatment plans.

The American Occupational Therapy Association defines occupational therapy as "a health and rehabilitation profession. Its practitioners provide services to individuals of all ages who have physical, developmental, emotional, and social deficits, and because of these conditions, need specialized assistance in learning skills to enable them to lead independent, productive, and satisfying lives."

The Differences Between P.T.s and O.T.s

P.T.s and O.T.s differ from each other in a few ways. Although they have the same goals, to make the patient as independent as possible, physical therapists deal only with the patients' physical difficulties. O.T.s work with physical and psychosocial aspects. A lot of occupational therapists work in psychiatric facilities, helping patients to cope with their emotional problems. Some patients have a combination of problems. They might have had a stroke, but are suffering from depression as well.

While they both deal with physical problems, they don't do it in the same way. An occupational therapist probably wouldn't help a person with ambulation skills, learning how to walk. However, both the physical and occupational therapist might focus on transfer skills, helping a person get from the bed to a chair, from the chair to a standing position.

EDUCATION
B.A./B.S. Required
Post Graduate Recommended

$$$ SALARY/EARNINGS
$30,000 to $75,000

JOB SETTINGS FOR PHYSICAL THERAPISTS

While those not in the know might think of physical therapists as working only in a hospital setting, there is, in actuality, a wide range of settings open to P.T. professionals. In addition to seeing patients in acute-care hospitals, both in- and out-patient, physical therapists see patients in their homes, providing home health care; in schools, working with students on the playing fields; in nursing homes; in rehab hospitals; in private practices; and in industry, doing job-site analyses, helping to prevent injuries. As an example, IBM or another large corporation could hire a physical therapist to evaluate risks the employees encounter, and then by taking the recommendations made by the physical therapist, they can redesign the workplace and lower their workmen's compensation payments.

Physical therapists can also travel, working for what is called a traveling company. This kind of company will make sure you are licensed in whatever state you might go to, and then they will send you around the country on temporary assignments, wherever there is a need.

Physical therapists work with the following patients or problems:

Premature infants

Pediatric patients

Obstetric patients

People with sports or traumatic injuries

People with birth or genetic defects

Adults with back or neck injuries

Stroke victims

Burn and wound victims

Amputees

Dancers and performing artists

Athletes

People with muscular sclerosis, Parkinson's disease, or neurological injuries

Post-op patients

Geriatric patients

TRAINING FOR PHYSICAL THERAPISTS

Physical therapists must have at least a bachelor's degree. Some go on for a master's and others earn their doctorate. Most schools require anywhere from 20 to 100 hours of observation time before future P.T.s can even apply to be admitted to a program. This observation time can be clocked while volunteering or working as a physical therapy aide.

Physical therapy programs can be found through the American Physical Therapy Association, whose address is listed at the end of this chapter.

Coursework covers mostly math and sciences as well as specific training on the techniques used in physical therapy, including exercise science and exercise physiology. Although the training is similar to that undertaken by personal trainers (the personal trainer occupation is covered in *On the Job: Real People Working in Service Businesses*), physical therapy training is more medically based. P.T. students study more pathology, doing cadaver dissections, for example. The study of anatomy and physiology is more extensive, as is muscle pathology. But the differences are explained easily by the different people each works with. Personal trainers deal with a healthy population for the most part; physical therapists work with patients who have disabilities or a variety of the other problems mentioned above.

EDUCATION
A.A./A.S. Required

$$$ SALARY/EARNINGS
$20,000 to $30,000

Physical Therapist Assistant

While the physical therapist is responsible for the design of treatment plans, the physical therapist assistant is trained to carry out those plans. Limitations for the physical therapist assistant are that they cannot update or change treatment plans.

Training for a physical therapist assistant career involves a two-year program ending with an associate's degree.

EDUCATION
H.S. Required
On-the-Job Training Possible

$$$ SALARY/EARNINGS
Minimum Wage to $12,000

Physical Therapy Aide

Physical therapy aides are usually trained on-the-job. They can't do direct patient care, but they help out the physical therapist and the physical therapist assistant. Aides might help a patient count the number of exercises he is doing, move equipment, bring patients to the treatment areas, or help a person walk or transfer from the bed to a chair.

SALARIES FOR THE PHYSICAL THERAPY PROFESSION

A brand new graduate physical therapist can make an excellent starting salary–between $35,000 to $40,000 a year, depending upon the region of the country in which he or she chooses to practice. Salaries go up with the number of years' experience.

Physical therapists working in home health can make $40 to $50 an hour and physical therapists in private practice can make between $85,000 and $100,000 a year. But these self-employed physical therapists have more expenses to cover, too, such as insurance. In private practice, a physical therapist has to wear many hats, one of which is that of bill collector. And it can be difficult sometimes to collect payments owed you.

Traveling physical therapists usually make a good hourly salary and have all their expenses covered, including flights, rental cars, hotel rooms, and meals.

Physical therapy assistants with a two-year degree can start out earning between $20,000 and $30,000 a year.

The non-professional position of physical therapy aide earns about $5 or so an hour.

JOB OUTLOOK FOR PHYSICAL THERAPISTS

The job outlook for physical therapists is excellent. There has been a shortage of physical therapists for quite a while now. There are two main reasons for this. The capabilities and problems that the physical therapist is qualified to handle have expanded, creating more of a demand.

Secondly, because academia doesn't pay well, there is a shortage of qualified people willing to teach in physical therapy training programs. When the teacher makes less money than the student, there is little motivation to follow that career path. Physical therapists with doctorates are required to teach master's and doctoral level students. The numbers of those qualified teachers are very low. Most physical therapists prefer to work in the field rather than in a classroom. With fewer teachers, fewer physical therapists can be trained, thus contributing to the shortage and increasing the demand.

EDUCATION
B.A./B.S. Required
Post Graduate Recommended

$$$ SALARY/EARNINGS
$30,000 to $40,000

JOB SETTINGS FOR OCCUPATIONAL THERAPISTS

O.T.s work with all types of patients, from the premature infant to geriatric patients, and see people with all kinds of diagnoses. This covers anything that would limit their ability to care for themselves–arthritis, hand injuries, burns, and neurological dysfunction, which takes in stroke patients and patients with MS or muscular dystrophy, cerebral palsy, brain tumors, and psychiatric problems.

O.T.s work in the following settings:

Acute care hospitals

Rehab hospitals

Psychiatric hospitals or wards

Pediatric hospitals or wards

Nursing homes

School systems

Private practice

TRAINING FOR OCCUPATIONAL THERAPISTS

Occupational therapists must earn a four-year degree, studying all the sciences–zoology, biology, physiology, anatomy, kinesiology. They also take psychology and abnormal psychology classes as well as child development, and study occupational therapy techniques.

After your four years, you will do a six- to nine-month internship, rotating in different kinds of facilities and specialties.

Once you pass your internship, you must pass a national exam to become a registered occupational therapist.

Specialties you can study are pediatrics, psychiatric, hands, and physical disabilities.

Some O.T.s go on for master's degrees, in occupational therapy or related fields such as administration or even physical therapy.

The personal qualities and skills you'll need to make a good O.T. are as follows:

You should be outgoing, with a lot of empathy, and a good sense of humor. You'll need to be open and willing to talk to your patients. You also have to be a good listener. Patients look at their therapists as someone they can talk to–doctors never have enough time for that kind of relationship. You also need good people skills, dealing with coworkers and the family members of your patients.

EDUCATION
A.A./A.S. Required

$$$ SALARY/EARNINGS
$20,000 to $30,000

Certified Occupational Therapy Assistants

Certified occupational therapy assistants study at a community college and earn a two-year associate's degree. Although they don't evaluate patients or make treatment plans, they function much as physical therapy assistants do, carrying out the plans.

Some universities have started weekend programs for O.T. assistants who want to go ahead and get their four-year degree. While they are employed full-time, they study every other weekend, finishing the bachelor's degree in about two years.

EDUCATION
H.S. Required
On-the-Job Training Possible

$$$ SALARY/EARNINGS
Minimum Wage to $12,000

Occupational Therapy Aides

Occupational therapy aides function similarly to their P.T. counterparts, helping the O.T.s and assistants with various duties.

SALARIES FOR THE OCCUPATIONAL THERAPY PROFESSION

Salaries for O.T.s are similar to those for physical therapists and can start at around an average of $35,000 a year. Starting salaries for certified occupational therapy assistants would average about $20,000 a year. Occupational therapy aides would earn from $5.00 to $5.50 an hour.

RELATED FIELDS

Others who work in the rehabilitation field include corrective therapists, recreational therapists, manual arts therapists, speech pathologists and audiologists, prosthetists, respiratory therapists, chiropractors, acupuncturists, and personal and athletic trainers.

INTERVIEW

Laurie DeJong
Physical Therapist

Laurie DeJong is assistant director of physical therapy at a large community hospital. She graduated in 1984 with a bachelor's degree in physical therapy from Quinnipiac College in Hamden, Connecticut.

What the Job's Really Like

"Physical therapists generally specialize, working in a particular setting or with certain kinds of patients. We evaluate patients, looking for pain, their flexibility or range of motion, their strength, and what kind of functional activities they do or need to do. For example, if the patient is a dancer, she needs to dance; if it's a child, she needs to play; if it's an adult, she needs to work, and so on. We do a complete evaluation, sitting down and talking to the patient about what the patient is looking for, about what we're looking for, and then, depending upon the person and her needs, we would design an appropriate treatment plan.

"Treatment plans generally include manual therapy, doing stretching or strengthening exercises, or specific joint mobilization exercises. We also use modalities such as hot packs, cold packs, ultrasound, or electric stimulation to help reduce pain.

"We do a lot of teaching, too, explaining the exercises to the patients, so they can carry on the activities at home without us. We do a lot of education in terms of posture and how patients can prevent their injuries from recurring. If our patients are children, we also work with the parents or teachers, how to do the exercises or how to best help the child function in the school arena. On the sports field we may be educating the coaches as to what kind of exercises a specific child needs.

"We also run classes, such as back schools, body awareness, or risk management, within the hospital and within industry.

"Part of the job is doing documentation–that's the part most of us don't like, but it's necessary.

"But it's a great profession to have. You can specialize in so many different areas. We all come out with a basic background and then you can tailor your expertise to the area you prefer.

"In my job I like the fact that I can do a lot of different things. We have a lot of hands-on time with our patients. We develop a treatment plan and then we see the patients generally two or three times a week for at least a month. I like working with the kids because I can see them for years. A child with developmental delays, such as cerebral palsy, for example, I'll see forever. We get to develop a rapport, spending time one-on-one with our patients. Doctors don't have the time to do that.

"I also like being able to keep up with the changes in health care, keeping myself on the cutting edge of what's happening out there.

"The stresses are the same as for everyone else. There's not enough time to do the job you have to do. It's also a challenge with the changes that are happening in health care. Some of the changes aren't fun and we don't like what's happening. There are now insurance companies telling us how we should treat our patients, as opposed to our dictating the kind of care our patients need. You'll find patients saying they know they need more treatment, but they won't be coming back to you because they can't afford it."

How Laurie DeJong Got Started

"I spent four years working in a rehab hospital and while there I started doing pediatrics and spent two years working with children as well as adults on an out-patient basis.

"For one year I had my own private practice doing home health and consultation in schools. I then moved to another state and joined the hospital as a staff physical therapist.

"I always liked medical things. I started playing hospital when I was about two. My parents told me I couldn't be a nurse, but I could become a doctor if I wanted to. But when I was 17 I realized how long it would take me to become a doctor. I learned about physical therapy from a guidance counselor, then realized that it would be the right career for me."

Expert Advice

"You have to really love working with people and you have to possess a great deal of patience. Change and improvement don't happen overnight. Often the person you're working with is impatient to get better, but you have to be the steadying force."

INTERVIEW
Helen Cox
Occupational Therapist

Helen Cox is an occupational therapy supervisor in the Rehab Services

Department of a community hospital.

What the Job's Really Like

"Occupational therapy is a health profession that helps people to do things for themselves within the limits of their disability or disease.

"First of all, we need to evaluate the patients to see what their skills are or where they have some deficits. Then we have to make a decision on whether we can improve those deficits. For instance, if someone has had a stroke, and they have a weak arm on the side of the stroke, do we feel we can, through exercise and other activities, improve the function of the arm and get it back to what it was prior to the stroke?

"We have to see if they have the motor ability, the muscle power, the strength to perform any activities. Do they have the coordination? Sometimes they might have the motor power but they couldn't pick up a coin from the table. That means they would be limited in doing some things for themselves.

"Sometimes in the evaluation, we realize that with arthritic patients, for example, they have lost the ability to manipulate small buttons. Then we can look into some adaptive equipment such as button hooks, dressing sticks, or elastic shoelaces, which don't need as fine a motor ability to use.

"After the assessment we set realistic goals with the patient. 'Where do you want to be functioning in a month? Where do you want to be functioning in three or four months?' The goals may be as simple as putting on socks or a sweater, or as long range as being able to sew or play the piano.

"When we have the goals, we use various activities, from putting round pegs in round holes to maybe even practicing the piano or using a computer keyboard. It depends on what skills they're trying to develop.

"At the end of 30 days we evaluate the progress. We may have initially measured grip and pinch strength and then we'll measure them again to see if there's been improvement.

"If we haven't reached the goals we look to see why. Maybe the patient had another stroke or something else interfered. If we do reach the goals, we make new short-term goals until the patient has reached his maximum potential.

"Being able to see people improve is the nicest part of the job. Sometimes patients surprise you with what they're able to accomplish."

How Helen Cox Got Started

"I originally planned to become a nurse, but while I was away at college, I was having problems with chemistry. My brother, who is a physical therapist, said to me, 'Why do you want to become a nurse, anyway, and work all those ridiculous hours on weekends, nights, and holidays?' My mom was a nurse and that's why I was pursuing it. My brother suggested I become an occupational therapist and I said, 'What's that?' He was working at a VA hospital, so I went there to visit the occupational therapy clinic. I saw that it was a lot of hands-on care and then I knew that that's what I wanted to do. I went to the University of Illinois in Chicago and earned my B.S. degree in occupational therapy in 1970."

Expert Advice

"A lot of people who think they want a career in the health professions consider becoming a doctor or a nurse the only options. But that couldn't be further from the truth. You need to understand what each area of the health professions does, then make your choice based on your own personality make-up."

• • •

FOR MORE INFORMATION

The following organization provides certification for personal trainers:

American College of Sports Medicine (ACSM)
Member and Chapter Services Department
P.O. Box 1440
Indianapolis, IN 46206

The following organization provides certification for personal trainers:

American Council on Exercise (ACE)
P.O. Box 910449
San Diego, CA 92191

American Occupational Therapy Association
P.O. Box 1725
1383 Piccard Drive
Rockville, MD 20849-1725

American Physical Therapy Association
1111 North Fairfax Street
Alexandria, VA 22314

American Therapeutic Recreation Association
c/o Associated Management Systems
P.O. Box 15215
Hattiesburg, MS 39402-5215

International Physical Fitness Association
415 W. Court Street
Flint, MI 48503

National Council for Therapeutic Recreation Certification
P.O. Box 479
Thiells, NY 10984-0479

National Therapeutic Recreation Society
2775 S. Quincy Street, Suite 300
Arlington, VA 22206-2204

CHAPTER 9 Speech-Language Pathologists and Audiologists

OVERVIEW

According to the American Speech-Language-Hearing Association (ASHA), speech and language disorders are "inabilities of individuals to understand and/or appropriately use the speech and language systems of society. Such disorders may range from simple sound repetitions or occasional miscalculations to the complete absence of the ability to use speech and language for communication."

For every 20 Americans who communicate "normally," there is one individual who is afflicted with a speech-language disorder. That numbers nearly 10 million people.

Hearing impairment ranges from the inability to hear speech and other sounds well and/or to understand speech even when it is heard, to the complete loss of any hearing.

Based on studies of a decade ago by the National Center for Health Statistics, it is estimated that hearing impairment in one or both ears affects approximately 2 out of every 100 school-age children; 29 out of every 100 people 65 years of age or older; and a total of 21.2 million Americans.

A career as a speech-language pathologist or audiologist offers an opportunity to help and interact with a wide variety of individuals, providing rewarding experiences for both the client and therapist. It is also a career for the researcher dedicated to finding new therapeutic approaches and technology.

⌂ EDUCATION
Post Graduate Required
Other

$$$ SALARY/EARNINGS
$30,000 to $75,000

Speech-Language Pathologists

A speech-language pathologist has a wide range of duties and choice of settings, age groups, and disorders with which to work. Speech-language pathologists screen, evaluate, and treat people with communication disorders. They also make referrals, provide counseling and instruction, supervise students and clinical fellows, teach, conduct research, and administer speech-language pathology programs.

Speech and language disorders can include the following:

• Disfluencies, including stuttering and other interruptions of normal speech flow, such as excessive hesitations, repeating the first sound in a word over and over, too frequently inserting extraneous syllables ("er," or "um,") or words and phrases into speech.

• Articulation disorders, substituting one sound for another ("free" instead of "three"), omitting a sound, or distorting a sound.

• Voice disorders, inappropriate pitch, quality, loudness, resonance, and duration.

• Aphasia, complete loss of speech (generally resulting from a stroke of head injury).

• Delayed language ability.

Those working in elementary schools spend a great deal of the time providing articulation therapy or phonologic therapy, teaching children to articulate more clearly. Some of the techniques they use involve playing games that have the child work with the same target sounds. Another technique is called auditory bombardment and it uses a set of headphones that amplifies the therapist's speech and plays it into the child's ear. The therapist reads a list of words that are amplified, helping the child focus on the correct sounds.

Another common disorder for speech-language pathologists to deal with is aphasia, an inability to either understand or produce speech due to a brain injury or brain disorder. This condition most commonly follows a stroke and sometimes follows brain trauma or accidents.

Although relying less heavily on devices than audiologists, speech-language pathologists do use equipment to check the health of vocal cords and detect any abnormal growths.

Audiologists

EDUCATION
Post Graduate Required
Other

$$$ SALARY/EARNINGS
$30,000 to $75,000

The primary functions of audiologists are to test hearing and to do rehabilitation work with hearing-impaired individuals and their significant others.

To test hearing and the functioning of the auditory system, audiologists use a range of electronic equipment, the audiometer and other devices for assessing performance of hearing aids. There are devices that plug into hearing aids and can be programmed to make the performance of the hearing aid appropriate for the hearing loss of that individual. There are also devices with very tiny microphones that are hooked up into tubes inserted directly into the ear canal to tell just how much sound is reaching the ear drum. Other devices test the functioning of a hearing aid independently of a person to make sure that all the electronics in the aid are working correctly.

The primary effect of a person's hearing loss is on the ability to communicate and the ability to hear speech. For most people, the most important person they want to be able to communicate with is their spouse or significant other. Therefore, therapy will focus not only on the hearing-impaired individual but on the spouse as well. Emphasis is placed on teaching good communication skills–everything from learning not to start a conversation from another room, to getting rid of other sources of noise by turning off the dishwasher or TV.

For people with more profound hearing loss, audiologists spend their time teaching the person to utilize what little hearing he or she has, working with other systems to help with speech, and teaching the person how to get along without hearing. Audiologists work with lip reading skills, sign language, and some simple devices such as a light in place of the doorbell, telephone, or alarm clock tones. The audiologist would have knowledge of these devices and be able to make them available to clients.

Communications Disorders Instructor

The old saying that 'those who can, do; those who can't, teach' doesn't apply here. In order for someone to become an instructor/professor in a university communication disorders program, he or she must have first become a certified speech-language pathologist or audiologist, and fulfilled all the requisite hours for practicing in the field. Those who return to the classroom after a stint in practice bring with them a wealth of hands-on experience in addition to their theoretical knowledge.

A Ph.D. is the usual requirement for entry into university teaching in a communication disorders program, as well as demonstrating an interest in guiding and supervising student therapists.

With such a nationwide shortage of certified speech-language pathologists and audiologists, the demand is on the increase for more teachers who can, in turn, train more qualified personnel.

Researchers

There are those who, rather than practice or teach, are more interested in a career in research. They are fascinated by the different problems human communication presents and work to find solutions to prevent, identify, assess, or rehabilitate speech, language, or hearing disorders.

Areas of interest for researchers include:

- Investigating the physical, biological, and physiological factors underlying normal communication.

- Exploring the impact of social, psychological, and psychophysiological factors on communication disorders.

- Cooperating with other professionals such as engineers, physicians, and educators to develop a comprehensive approach to working with people with communication disorders.

Researchers are most often affiliated with universities and divide their time between classroom teaching and working on various research questions. The usual requirement for a research scientist is a minimum of a Ph.D. degree.

Some research scientists work in industrial settings, for pharmaceutical companies or for manufacturers of hearing aids or computers.

JOB SETTINGS

Medical Clinics and Hospitals

Therapists working in a medical clinic or hospital setting come in contact with a wide variety of people with a wide variety of disorders. They are able to establish close relationships with their clients because they work with them over a period of time. The relationship usually begins from the point before they've had the cause of the disorder diagnosed, through the diagnosis, and treatment and therapy.

Therapists in this setting also get to work closely with other professionals–physicians, nurses, in some cases neurology professionals, psychologists, physical therapists–to collaborate on effective treatment plans.

Nursing Homes/Rehab Centers

In this setting therapists work with elderly patients or patients who have recovered enough from their stroke or injury to be released from the hospital, but are not yet independent enough to return home. Work duties consist mainly of diagnosing and carrying out treatment plans.

Public and Private Schools

Here the speech-language pathologist works with children, most commonly treating them in a group situation. Children with similar problems would be excused from their regular classrooms for an hour, two or three times a week, to work on particular speech disorders.

Some speech-language pathologists are based at one school; others travel to several different schools within the district.

In a school setting, screening for hearing impairment is usually done by the school nurse; the audiologist works more with diagnosis and therapy.

State Schools for the Deaf and Similar Institutions

Here therapists work with a more narrow range of problems. Students would all be deaf or perhaps deaf and blind. Students and therapists would meet on a more regular basis than in public or private school settings and the work would focus mainly on improving speech skills.

Working with completely deaf children or deaf and blind children is by far the most challenging–and for some the most rewarding–area of the communication disorders field.

Private Practice

Speech-language pathologists and audiologists can carve out an excellent career for themselves in private practice. Their services are covered by insurance and they can visit clients in their homes or set up their own offices and take referrals from hospitals, ENT (ear, nose, and throat) specialists, and other professionals in the medical community.

Because the schools don't have enough staff to see all the students they have identified with communication disorders, private practitioners also receive referrals through the school board. During the summer months when schools are closed, parents might take their child to a private practice speech-language pathologist to carry on the therapy started during the regular school year.

Home Health Care Agencies

Home health care agencies operate on both local and national levels. A therapist or audiologist signed up with a local agency will be given assignments as requests come in. National agencies are used by hospitals and other concerns all over the country and provide an opportunity for a practitioner to travel to different cities on short- or long-term assignments.

Colleges and Universities

Some experienced speech-language pathologists and audiologists choose to work in an academic setting, teaching students preparing for careers in communication disorders or conducting research.

TRAINING AND QUALIFICATIONS

Just as with other communications programs, programs in speech-language pathology and audiology can be housed in a number of different university departments with a number of different names and degrees conferred. Commonly, programs are called communication disorders, communicative disorders, communication science, speech communications, speech pathology, and speech-language and hearing pathology. The program name preferred by ASHA is Communication Sciences and Disorders. Degrees conferred could be a Master of Science, Master of Arts, or Master of Education.

The American Speech-Language-Hearing Association certifies speech-language pathologists and audiologists who have met certain criteria. To become certified and awarded a Certificate of Clinical Competence in Speech-Language Pathology (CCC-SLP) or a Certificate of Competence in Audiology (CCC-A), or certificates in both areas, candidates must:

- Earn a master's degree covering the requisite number of credit hours from an institution whose program is accredited by the Educational Standard Board of the American Speech-Language-Hearing Association.

- Complete the requisite number of hours in a supervised clinical observation and a supervised clinical practicum. The practicum cannot be undertaken until sufficient coursework for such an experience has been completed.

- Complete a Clinical Fellowship of at least 36 weeks of full-time professional experience or its part-time equivalent in a variety of settings.

The master's degree in speech pathology and audiology entails at least 350 hours of clinical contact with patients or clients with communication disorders.

Following the master's program, the final step in completing certification is the successful participation in and completion of a clinical fellowship year. Often the first nine months of your job working full-time can be considered as your clinical fellowship year. During that time you would have a certified speech-language pathologist supervising your work. If you were working only half-time, it would take you longer to complete the clinical fellowship year.

The clinical fellowship gives you a chance to integrate all you have learned through coursework and the clinical practicum.

Bachelor's degree programs are available in communication disorders and many have coursework designed to mesh with a master's program. However, a B.A. in speech-language pathology or communication disorders is not required to enter a master's program in speech-language pathology.

Because of the shortage of certified communication disorders specialists, some bachelor's level pathologists do find work. The only setting in which they can be employed with just a bachelor's degree is within different public school systems in some states. They must, however, sign a contract promising to get their master's within four to seven years.

They are allowed to work toward the master's while they are employed, but that can be problematic. Most people working within the public schools are on duty during the times that graduate courses are offered. There are some night courses available, but in some states the programs are not currently designed to accommodate the schedule of working students.

In addition to the coursework, you need between 350 and 375 contact hours in a practicum experience, some of which must be acquired in several different settings working with different types of disorders and different age groups. If you are in the public schools the logistics become very difficult.

Some employed B.A.-level pathologists take a sabbatical from their job to be able to finish their master's degree. Most find going straight for the master's degree without working to be the most efficient method.

ASHA publishes a handbook that specifies the exact requirements for professional certification. You can contact them at the address listed at the end of this chapter.

Currently there are 39 states that legally require individuals who engage in private practice or who work in nonpublic agencies to hold a license in speech-language pathology or audiology. Generally, the requirements are similar to those for ASHA certification.

ASHA maintains a list of all state licensing boards and of all accredited university programs in speech-language pathology and audiology.

JOB OUTLOOK

Projections are that job openings will outstrip the supply of qualified candidates for the next ten years. The American Speech-Language-Hearing Association (ASHA) in 1994 prepared a report announcing that shortages of speech-language pathologists and audiologists continue, especially in school settings.

The American Hospital Association (AHA) reports chronic shortages in key hospital occupations including speech-language pathologists. In 1991 one out of every ten speech-language pathologist positions remained unfilled and the vacancies continue.

This is all very good news for future speech-language pathologists and audiologists. Not only are plum jobs waiting for you upon graduation, money is now available to see you through training. In an attempt to meet the need for more trained professional, scholarship programs have been set up throughout the country on local and state levels as well as through individual university graduate programs. Some of these programs guarantee employment upon graduation.

To find out more about the various scholarships that are available, check with ASHA, local school boards, or through graduate communication disorders programs at universities.

SALARIES FOR SPEECH-LANGUAGE PATHOLOGISTS AND AUDIOLOGISTS

Because of the shortage of certified speech-language pathologists and audiologists mentioned earlier, salaries in this career path are very good and are on the rise. The American Speech-Language-Hearing Association (ASHA) conducts an annual salary survey of its members. The most current figures available at this writing are reported from 1993 earnings, which show a 2.9 percent increase from 1992 for certified speech-language pathologists and a 3.4 percent increase from 1992 for audiologists. The median annual salary for speech-language pathologists in 1992 was $34,000 and in 1993 was $35,000. Audiologists earned a median annual salary of $35,782 in 1992 and $37,000 in 1993.

Here are a few other points to consider about salaries in this field:

- Salaries could jump from $28,000 or $30,000 up to $40,000 to $45,000 after the clinical fellowship year, depending upon where you work.

- After a few years salaries could go to $60,000 or higher.

- Speech-language pathologists or audiologists working in a school system are usually paid on the same scale as teachers.

- According to a survey conducted by the American Hospital Association, more than 70 percent of the hospitals polled reported that the lack of available candidates is the greatest deterrent to successful recruitment. Hospital human resources executives said that raising salaries is their most common recruitment and retention technique.

- Salaries for college and university instructors and professors generally run much lower than those working in the field. It is not unusual for a professor to see a new student graduate and land a job paying more than he or she is earning.

RELATED FIELDS

Workers in other rehabilitation occupations include occupational therapists, physical therapists, recreational therapists, and rehabilitation counselors.

INTERVIEW
Fay Dudley
Speech-Language Pathologist

Fay Dudley is a speech-language pathologist and is also the supervisor of the speech-language pathology department at a small community hospital. She has been in the field for close to 15 years.

What the Job's Really Like

"I work with adult neurological patients and voice patients, primarily. In addition I do administrative work.

"The neurological patients have had damage, usually as a result of a stroke or hemorrhage or a head trauma of some sort. The voice patients range from people who have been diagnosed with cancer and have had their larynx removed, or they have vocal cord nodules or polyps, or just general vocal cord abuse. These patients talk a lot or talk quickly and emphatically, or are smokers.

"I work Monday through Friday, 8 to 4:30. I spend between 30 minutes to an hour with each patient, depending on what the patient can tolerate and what he requires. I probably see five or six patients a day. Then I do the administrative work the rest of the time. I have three other speech-language pathologists whom I supervise and, occasionally, we hire per diem therapists, therapists who come in on an as-needed basis, depending on how busy the caseload is.

"I treat outpatients the majority of the time, but if we're short on staff, I'll treat inpatients, too.

"When a patient has actually followed through with my suggestions and I can see progress or hear the changes, that's the most rewarding part of my job.

"And we're lucky enough here to get state-of-the-art equipment related to voice. One of the newest things in the field is doing something called videostroboscopy. You can observe how an individual's vocal cords function and actually see the movement of the cords. And you're also videotaping it at the same time, so you have a record for documentation and review purposes.

"With all the new equipment you can increase your knowledge base and learn. Because, otherwise, if you've been in the field for an extensive period of time, burnout can set in.

"The work, at times, can get monotonous. Once you know the job well, some things are so rote, you don't even have to think about them. When you get an exciting case or something that's different or you're unfamiliar with it, that's great. But most of the cases you get day in and day out are the same. And you get bored.

"As a result, some people leave the field, or sometimes they just accept that it's part and parcel of the job. And there are always times when it's worse, and times when it's better. To keep it interesting you just have to try to expand your horizons or get into new areas of the field. You can work in a different setting or with a different population. One of the things we do that's different is occasionally we work with foreign accent reduction. But we don't get much call for it because it's considered cosmetic and it's not covered by insurance. And therapy is expensive."

How Fay Dudley Got Started

"I had been in business before, in a position where I made decisions and handed decisions down, but there wasn't too much people contact. The main component that led me to this profession was having a lot of people contact and being able to help people.

"I also had a niece who was deaf from meningitis at nine months of age and so that got me thinking about deaf education or speech pathology. I started reading on the subject and thought everything was interesting and that maybe I could get into that.

"I went to the University of Connecticut for a semester on a nondegree status to take some basic courses and to see if I liked it. I already had a bachelor's degree in French and political science, so I went for a master's in speech-language pathology in 1979 and I finished in 1981.

"I ended up working for a corporation that had several contracts with nursing homes. I worked in Pennsylvania with them for two years, then I opened up the Florida division for them. In 1985 I joined the staff of a community hospital. In 1993 I was promoted to supervisor."

Expert Advice

"You need to want to work with people, but you have to recognize that there is emotional stress involved. You have patients who make progress and patients who don't. Some patients you can get involved with and if they don't progress, it's so frustrating for them. You can definitely sympathize with them because you see that frustration. And that can be emotionally draining on you.

"Overall, I think it's a good field and I've enjoyed it. Again, I think that's because I haven't been stagnant, I've been able to do various things in it. It helps to be independent and organized. If you have that quest for knowledge it will help you stay in the field.

"To know if it's really the field for you, it helps to do observation. Actually go in and watch a speech therapist do therapy. And see a variety of cases, children and adults.

"To find someone you can observe, you can call the national organization or call a local hospital, or even look in the Yellow Pages under speech-language pathology. Check out the different settings. More often than not, whoever's in charge is very willing and open for someone to come in and observe."

● ● ●

FOR MORE INFORMATION

ASHA is the main professional association for speech-language pathologists and audiologists. It has over 67,000 members and certificate holders and recognizes 52 state speech and hearing association affiliates.

It provides certification to qualified speech-language pathologists and audiologists and accreditation to qualifying university programs.

American Speech-Language-Hearing Association (ASHA)
10801 Rockville Pike
Rockville, MD 20852

Council for Better Hearing and Speech Month
1616 H Street, NW
Washington, DC 20006

National Student Speech-Language-Hearing Association
10801 Rockville Pike
Rockville, MD 20852

Telecommunications for the Deaf
8719 Colesville Rd. #300
Silver Spring, MD 20910

Chapter 10 Dentists

EDUCATION
Post Graduate Required

$$$ SALARY/EARNINGS
$75,000+

OVERVIEW

Dentists diagnose, prevent, and treat problems of the teeth and tissues of the mouth. They remove decay and fill cavities, examine x-rays, place protective plastic sealants on children's teeth, straighten teeth, and repair fractured teeth.

They also perform corrective surgery of the gums and supporting bones to treat gum diseases. Dentists extract teeth and make molds and measurements for dentures to replace missing teeth. Dentists provide instruction in diet, brushing, flossing, the use of fluorides, and other aspects of dental care, as well.

They also administer anesthetics and write prescriptions for antibiotics and other medications.

Most dentists are solo practitioners, that is, they own their own businesses and work alone or with a small staff. Some dentists have partners, and a few work for other dentists as associate dentists.

Specialties

Most dentists are general practitioners who handle a wide variety of dental needs. Other dentists practice in one of eight specialty areas.

Orthodontists, the largest group of specialists, straighten teeth.
Oral and maxillofacial surgeons, the next largest group, operate on the mouth and jaws.

The remainder specialize in:

Pediatric dentistry, dentistry for children.
Periodontics, treating the gums and the bone supporting the teeth.
Prosthodontics, making artificial teeth or dentures.
Endodontics, root canal therapy.
Dental public health.
Oral pathology, studying diseases of the mouth.

TRAINING

To practice dentistry, all dentists must be licensed. To qualify for a license in most states, a candidate must graduate from a dental school accredited by the American Dental Association's Commission on Dental Accreditation and pass written and practical examinations. Candidates may fulfill the written part of the state licensing by passing the National Board Dental Examinations. Individual states or regional testing agencies give the written and/or practical examinations.

Currently, about 15 states require dentists to obtain a specialty license before practicing as a specialist. Requirements include two to four years of post-graduate education and, in some cases, completion of a special state examination. Most state licenses permit dentists to engage in both general and specialized practice.

Dentists who want to teach or do research usually spend an additional two to five years in advanced dental training in programs operated by dental schools or hospitals.

Dental schools require a minimum of two years of college-level predental education. However, most dental students have at least a bachelor's degree. Predental education includes courses in both the sciences and humanities.

All dental schools require applicants to take the Dental Admissions Test (DAT). Dental school usually takes four years.

Most dental schools award the degree of Doctor of Dental Surgery (D.D.S.). The rest award an equivalent degree, Doctor of Dental Medicine (D.M.D.).

SALARIES

The net median income of dentists in private practice was about $90,000 a year in 1992, according to the American Dental Association. Net median income of those in specialty practices was about $130,000 a year, and for those in general practice, $85,000 a year. Dentists in the beginning years of their practice often earn less, while those in mid-career earn more.

A relatively large proportion of dentists are self-employed. Like other business owners, these dentists must provide their own health insurance, life insurance, and retirement benefits.

RELATED FIELDS

Dentists examine, diagnose, prevent, and treat diseases and abnormalities. So do clinical psychologists, optometrists, physicians, chiropractors, veterinarians, and podiatrists.

INTERVIEW
David Kagan
Dentist

David Kagan has been a general dentist since 1983. He recently moved into new office space and plans to bring another dentist on board. He employs two dental assistants, two hygienists, two front administrators/receptionists, a high school student, and a periodontist who comes in on an as-needed basis.

What the Job's Really Like

"What I like to do is preventive dentistry. My favorite thing about being a dentist is that 99 percent of what happens in dentistry, the problems people have, is already known, predictable, and preventable. What I consider preventive dentistry to be starts with little kids, making sure they get fluoride, proper home care instruction, sealants put on their teeth. With adults I try to do dentistry that will have the least likelihood of ever needing to be replaced or done again at a later date.

"I also like cosmetic dentistry. There's a lot cosmetic dentistry can do for someone, helping them dramatically, with relatively conservative type procedures, such as bleaching their teeth or using porcelain veneers.

"If my patients are already healthy, I like to be able to keep them that way. If they're not healthy, I like to try to get them that way. I have two hygienists and will probably be getting a third sometime soon.

"We're very periodontally aware, too, making sure that the gums and bones stay healthy in people. I'm also very much into high tech; that's a big hobby of mine. In 1987 I got my first intra-oral camera to show patients what is actually going on in their teeth. Right now, I'm also using a needleless anesthesia and a machine that does cavity preparation without drilling.

"And I'm very much into learning about dentistry and keeping current. I've spent a ton of time and money on continuing education for myself and my staff.

"I don't think I'm a typical dentist. For example, I hate doing crowns and bridges, but most dentists love to do that. Although these procedures are necessary, the reason people need them is generally because of a lack of proper care over an extended period of time. But no matter how good a dentist I am, I might not have the capability of influencing them to change the pattern that created those problems. My work may be for naught and I don't like that feeling. I like things to be very predictable. And the materials I choose to work with, cast gold, for example, require more time and skill. But the results are longer lasting and I'm willing to put in the time.

"Most people who become dentists are technical, scientific type people. Maybe that's a left brain type of person. So the hardest thing for me, though it can be the most fun, too, is dealing with people.

"The average dental education of a lay person is so pathetically low, and this is a fault of dentistry. Dentists don't educate patients the way they need to be educated. They drill, fill, and bill.

"And most people shop dentistry the way I would shop for an appliance. They call up and ask for prices on different procedures. I don't look at dentistry that way; I look at the mouth as an organ like your heart is. And if you start messing around with it, you're going to have trouble your whole life. I try to prevent that kind of trouble. But it's frustrating getting the patients to a level where they understand what we're trying to do.

"The gratifying thing is when you're able to take someone and turn them around. They follow through, they improve, and they appreciate what you've done for them."

How David Kagan Got Started

"When I was five years old I knew I wanted to be a dentist. Other kids thought they wanted to be firemen or cowboys, but I never wanted to be anything other than a dentist. I think the original seed was just there, almost like a calling.

"What got me into it when I got older was that both my parents are involved in science. My father is a chemist and my mother is a pharmacist. I was always interested in science in school and I wanted to have a job where I could help people. I also liked the medical idea, but I didn't want to have the life or death type of situations.

"When I was growing up my father only gave me one bit of advice, and that was to be your own boss. Being a dentist fit in well with that.

"I went to Muhlenberg College for two years, then transferred to the University of Maryland in College Park and graduated in 1979 with a B.S. in microbiology. Then I went to the University of Medicine and Dentistry of New Jersey and graduated in 1983 with a D.M.D. I took some boards and decided I wanted to be in Florida. I worked in Tallahassee for a while but found out the guy I was working for was involved in some sort of Medicaid fraud, so I was out of there.

"I moved to the West Palm Beach area and worked in ten or so different places as a salaried dentist, just getting enough days in. I was paid by commission, a percentage of what I took in. I did that for two years, then I heard through a family member about a dentist who wanted to sell his practice. Borrowing all the money from a variety of places, eventually, in 1985, I was able to buy it from him."

Expert Advice

"You'll never really know what it's like until you actually do it. And not only that, you probably won't like what you do until you're good at it. So, unless you have some sort of a natural talent, you'll have to work hard at this before you enjoy it.

"And although you have to take science courses, you don't have to like physics or math to be a dentist. There are so many different areas to go into, you could like so many different things. Find out your area and work at it."

●   ●   ●

FOR MORE INFORMATION

For information on dentistry as a career and a list of accredited dental schools, contact:

SELECT Program
Department of Career Guidance
American Dental Association
211 E. Chicago Ave.
Chicago, IL 60611

American Association of Dental Schools
1625 Massachusetts Ave., NW
Washington, DC 20036

The American Dental Association also will furnish a list of state boards of dental examiners. Persons interested in practicing dentistry should obtain the requirements for licensure from the board of dental examiners of the state where they plan to work.

For information on scholarships, grants, and loans, including federal financial aid, prospective dental students should contact the office of student financial aid at the schools to which they apply.

CHAPTER 11 Optometrists

🎓 **EDUCATION**
Post Graduate Required

💲💲💲 **SALARY/EARNINGS**
$40,000 to $75,000+

OVERVIEW

Over half the people in the United States wear glasses or contact lenses. Optometrists (doctors of optometry, also known as O.D.s) provide most of the primary vision care people need.

Optometrists examine people's eyes to diagnose vision problems and eye disease. They treat vision problems, and in most statesthey treat certain eye diseases, such as conjunctivitis or corneal infections, as well.

Optometrists use instruments and observation to examine eye health and to test patients' visual acuity, depth and color perception, and their ability to focus and coordinate the eyes. They analyze test results and develop a treatment plan.

Optometrists prescribe eyeglasses, contact lenses, vision therapy, and low vision aids. They use drugs for diagnosis in all states, and, as of 1993, they may use topical and oral drugs to treat some eye diseases in 37 states.

Most optometrists are in general practice. Some specialize in work with the elderly, with children, or with partially sighted persons who use specialized visual aids. Some specialize in contact lenses, sports vision, or vision therapy. A few teach optometry or do research.

Most optometrists are private practitioners who also handle the business aspects of running an office, such as developing a patient base, hiring employees, keeping records, and ordering equipment and supplies. Optometrists who operate franchise optical stores may also have some of these duties.

Although many optometrists are in solo practice, a growing number are in partnership or group practice. Some optometrists work as salaried employees of other optometrists or of ophthalmologists. Others work in hospitals, health maintenance organizations (HMOs), or retail optical stores.

Ophthalmologists and Opticians

Optometrists should not be confused with ophthalmologists or dispensing opticians. Ophthalmologists are physicians who diagnose and treat eye diseases and injuries. They perform surgery and prescribe drugs. Like optometrists, they also examine eyes and prescribe eyeglasses and contact lenses. Dispensing opticians fit and adjust eyeglasses and in some states may fit contact lenses according to prescriptions written by ophthalmologists or optometrists.

TRAINING FOR OPTOMETRISTS

All states require that optometrists be licensed. Applicants for a license must have a Doctor of Optometry degree from an accredited optometry school and pass both a written and a clinical state board examination. In many states, applicants can substitute the examinations of the National Board of Examiners in Optometry, usually taken during the student's academic career, for part or all of the written examination. Licenses are renewed every one to two years and in most states, continuing education credits are needed for renewal.

To complete the Doctor of Optometry degree you must complete a four-year program at an accredited optometry school preceded by at least three years of preoptometric study at an accredited college or university (most optometry students hold a bachelor's degree).

Applicants must take the Optometry Admissions Test (OAT), which measures academic ability and scientific comprehension. Most applicants take the test after their sophomore or junior year. Competition for admission is keen.

One-year postgraduate clinical residency programs are available for optometrists who wish to specialize in family practice, optometry, pediatric optometry, geriatric optometry, low vision rehabilitation, vision therapy, contact lenses, hospital-based optometry, and primary care optometry.

SALARIES

Incomes vary depending upon location, specialization, and other factors. Salaried optometrists tend to earn more initially than optometrists who set up their own independent practice, because of the cost of the initial outlay. In the long run, however, those in private practice generally earn more.

According to the American Optometric Association, new optometry graduates in their first year of practice earn an average income of about $45,000. Overall, optometrists earn an average of about $75,000.

RELATED FIELDS

Workers in other occupations who apply scientific knowledge to prevent, diagnose, and treat disorders and injuries are chiropractors, dentists, physicians, podiatrists, veterinarians, speech-language pathologists, and audiologists

INTERVIEW

Ronie Zaruches
Optometrist

Dr. Ronie Zaruches is an independent optometrist and has maintained two offices for the past five years. He has been in practice since 1985.

What the Job's Really Like

"The optometrist is considered the gatekeeper to eye care. They're the primary doctor patients usually see before specialty care. They can pick up high blood pressure changes, diabetic changes, and all sorts of things by evaluating the retina and the health of the eye.

"In a typical day in my office, patients come in and complete a form that includes a comprehensive health and medical history, any medications being used, and any visual problems. In the exam room I find out why they're here. Do they need a new prescription? Did they break their glasses? Are they having problems seeing far away or close up? Do they need contacts? Or do they have an eye infection?

"I perform the exam, checking vision, eye movement, checking the prescription with certain equipment, evaluating the external part of the eye with a microscope. I do glaucoma testing and evaluate the health of the retina.

"In the majority of states now, optometrists can treat some eye problems with drops and I can prescribe topical medication, but I cannot do any invasive procedure. So, if someone were to come in with, for argument's sake, a little piece of metal chip or wood chip in the eye, that I could remove because that's considered external. But I can't do any cataract or retinal surgery. I can treat eye infections or abrasions but if I notice, for example, diabetic changes I pick up during my examination, changes that I feel would need any type of surgical procedure or additional evaluation, then I would refer the patient to an ophthalmologist.

"I like the patient interaction, but I enjoy the pathology and the health evaluation portion the most, mainly because I like medicine. If I find pathology, I'm not happy for the patient, but I'm happy that I picked it up and was able to refer them to the proper source for treatment.

"The refraction portion, getting the eyeglass prescription, gets a bit monotonous after a while—I have no qualms about it but it's the least interesting.

"I enjoy what I do, I like it a lot, but the field is changing so much. It's frustrating in the sense that I wish I would have had my own practice. But when you get out of school, you owe a bundle on student loans–I've been paying for ten years.

"It's a huge expense to start your own practice. I don't own the optical end, making lenses, selling frames. I get a fee per each exam and a fee for contacts.

"This way, leasing space from an optical setup, all the equipment is provided. It's a big outlay, starting your own practice–all the equipment, and you have to stock about $20,000 worth of frames. Then there's advertising, rent, remodeling. So down the road, once the loans are paid off, it could be an option."

How Ronie Zaruches Got Started

"I was an art student at Brooklyn College, but in the practical world you have to make money and I wasn't going to be able to do that with art. So after graduating college, I ended up working on Wall Street for about a year and a half doing securities research. But even there I was making very little money and I decided I wanted to be my own boss.

"I've always been into anatomy, because everything I did with art revolved around that. I checked into the possibility of dental school, medical school, podiatry, and optometry. I decided I wanted to be in a, more or less, normal profession where I would have normal hours and wouldn't be on call all the time. So I eliminated medicine. But still, I didn't have enough of a background for the other fields and I had to go back to college for a year and a half to take all the science courses I needed.

"During that period, I observed what podiatrists and optometrists did, sat down with them and watched them do exams and that sort of thing. Optometry seemed the most interesting.

"After obtaining all my requirements and taking the admissions test for optometry school, I got accepted to the Pennsylvania School of Optometry in Philadelphia and graduated with an O.D. and another bachelor's degree in 1985.

"I was a salaried employee of a group practice for a while in New Jersey then, basically, I became an independent contractor and practiced for a variety of offices in New York. Now I maintain two offices, leasing space from a group of opticians."

Expert Advice

"Five years ago I probably would have said it's a great career. Now that medicine in general is changing so drastically, it's not what it used to be—especially with Managed Care programs, cutting costs across the board for health care. Doctors are getting paid less money for supposedly the same quality of care, and it's very difficult now to make the same living you might have made five or ten years ago.

"Another factor is all these price clubs, which sell their products–contacts, frames–below cost. This makes for a lot of competition for the solo optometrist.

"I would suggest you reconsider most areas of medicine as a career. If I were to go back to school right now, I'd choose radiology. They make the most money, and it's the nicest lifestyle. Sure, the things you see are life threatening, but you're evaluating them and reporting your findings to other doctors.

"If you really want to be an optometrist, I think it could be a nice career. You can make a decent living, though you won't get rich, unless you have significant money to invest."

●   ●   ●

FOR MORE INFORMATION

For information on optometry as a career, and a listing of accredited optometric educational institutions, as well as required preoptometry courses, write to:

American Optometric Association
Educational Services
243 North Lindbergh Blvd.
St. Louis, MO 63141-7881

The Board of Optometry in each state can supply information on licensing requirements.

For information on specific admission requirements and sources of financial aid, contact the admissions officer of individual optometry schools.

CHAPTER 12 Pharmacists

🎓 EDUCATION
B.A./B.S. Required
Post Graduate Recommended

$$$ SALARY/EARNINGS
$40,000 to $75,000

OVERVIEW

Pharmacists dispense drugs prescribed by physicians and other health practitioners and provide helpful information to customers about their use. They also advise doctors and other health practitioners on the selection, dosages, side effects, and contraindications of medications.

Job Settings

A pharmacist has a number of settings from which to choose–hospitals, HMOs, or retail pharmacies, including chain stores, independent pharmacies, discount and supermarket concessions.

Those working in hospitals dispense medication and advise the medical staff on the selection and effects of drugs, in some cases making rounds with them, checking on and monitoring patients.

Pharmacists in retail settings advise customers about prescription and over-the-counter medication. Those who own or manage a pharmacy may buy and sell non-health-related products, hire and supervise personnel, and oversee the general operation of the pharmacy.

TRAINING

To become a pharmacist you must graduate from an accredited college of pharmacy, pass a state exam, and participate in an internship supervised by a licensed pharmacist.

Five years of study are required beyond a high school diploma, resulting in a B.S. in pharmacy, the degree received by most graduates. This degree is generally accepted for positions in community pharmacies, but more and more hospital pharmacies are requiring a Pharm.D. or Doctorate of Pharmacy. A sixth year of study will earn you this degree. If you already hold a bachelor's degree, you may enter a Pharm.D. course, but the combined number of years of study is usually longer than six years.

Admission requirements to pharmacy programs vary. Some will accept students directly from high school; others expect one or two years of college level prepharmacy education. This can be obtained at a community college. Some colleges require the student take the P-CAT, or Pharmacy College Admissions Test. You should study mathematics and basic sciences such as chemistry, biology, and physics, as well as courses in the humanities and social sciences.

Once you are licensed, many states expect you to take a certain number of continuing education credits per year to keep that license active.

SALARIES

The following table shows excerpts from a survey conducted by *Drug Topics* magazine, published by Medical Economics Publishing, Inc.

Setting	Average Base Salary
Independent drug stores	$45,300
Chain drug stores	$49,800
Hospitals	$50,300
Supermarkets	$51,200
HMOs	$52,300
Discount stores	$53,200

Median annual salaries of full-time salaried pharmacists were $45,000. The lowest 10 percent earned less than $26,100 and the top 10 percent more than $59,500.

The survey also showed that pharmacists employed in the West earned more than pharmacists in other regions of the country. It also revealed that pharmacists employed by chains, supermarkets, discount stores, and HMOs receive more benefits than those employed by independent drug stores.

Pharmacists who own their own pharmacies often can earn much more than salaried pharmacists. However, independent pharmacists also run the risk of going under, just as with any other kind of business enterprise.

EDUCATION
H.S. Required
On-the-Job Training Possible
A.A./A.S. Recommended

$$$ SALARY/EARNINGS
$12,000 to $20,000

Pharmacy Assistants/Technicians

Pharmacy technicians and/or assistants mix pharmaceutical preparations, dispense medications, label and store supplies, all under the supervision of a licensed pharmacist. They might also be responsible for cleaning equipment and work areas.

Training is often on-the-job, though now a few community colleges across the country are offering one- and two-year programs in this area.

RELATED FIELDS

Other professionals who also work with pharmaceutical compounds are pharmaceutical chemists and pharmacologists. Others who are knowledgeable about pharmaceuticals can work as sales representatives for pharmaceutical companies.

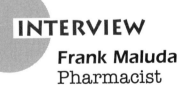

INTERVIEW
Frank Maluda
Pharmacist

In 1985, after working for five years for a major chain, Frank Maluda became independent and bought Romano's Pharmacy, a neighborhood operation in Coral Springs, Florida. He has about 10 to 12 employees–two part-time pharmacists, one full-time pharmacy technician, one full-time stock manager/front store manager, several clerks, and a post office substation for which he supplies the personnel.

He works 48 to 50 hours, six days a week. Forty-two of those hours are spent filling prescriptions, the remainder is designated for paperwork.

What the Job's Really Like

"To be a pharmacist and to own your own business you have to be a jack-of-all-trades, or you need to recognize what you don't know so you can hire someone who does know.

"Working for a chain, you have a front store manager, and the pharmacist is the pharmacy manager. You're spoon fed, so to speak, with Plan-O-Grams (marketing tools) given to you, with help with the computer provided. As an independent, you do it all yourself.

"And when you're in a chain, you don't have as many drug reps coming in to see you, it's done at the corporate level. But in an independent pharmacy, they come in to give you information about new drugs and you can get bombarded with all of this. It can put you off. But they do have a lot of information and it's part of your continuing education right there. They give you a lot of material and can even supply you with your continuing education credits.

"A big part of the business is done over the phone. You can start with a doctor's office calling in a prescription, then you transcribe it onto a prescription pad, enter it into the computer, print out labels and information sheets for the customers. Then you count out the medication. It can be done by hand or by machine. Personally, I feel with the cleaning and all the maintenance of this machinery, it doesn't justify my need for it in a retail setting. I do it by hand.

"The most important role is trying to prevent drug interactions, and the computer helps with that. The software tracks your customers' previous prescriptions and will check for adverse drug interactions. You also have to rely on your own medical knowledge gained from your experience in pharmacy. And it's also knowing your customer.

"A lot of questions get asked about the different disease states. 'What is my prognosis? What other treatments are there?' Quite often they feel funny talking to their doctor and feel more comfortable and more at ease discussing their concerns with their pharmacist.

"And it's nice that we have a good library of reference books behind us to fall back on. You can't answer every question off the top of your head.

"Another part of the job is dealing with doctors. Sometimes they'll call us and say, 'Hey, I've got a patient who has this type of bacteria diagnosed. What antibiotic is it sensitive to?' I'd either know the answer or have handbooks at my disposal that would give me quicker access to the information than the doctor has. Doctors also call up and ask about the costs of drugs and the ones that cost less for their patients who are watching their pennies. They also ask about the generic alternatives. That's also a very important role of the pharmacist, to offer the generic and let it be known that there would be a cost savings. But with generics, there are times when it's appropriate and times when it isn't. I would lay off generics if it meant the heart or a psychological type medication or sustained release medication, like a cold capsule or diet suppressant. The latter are hard to duplicate, the characteristics and the way the drug is dispensed. And the FDA complicates matters in that they will pass a drug as okay to sell if it is found to be 80 percent as effective as the brand name. But 80 percent is a big leeway. I make sure I let my customers know that.

"Another thing pharmacists have to be on the lookout for is fraudulent prescriptions. If we suspect something, we'll call the doctor's office and verify if they just called in. Or we check their service or ask if a Mr. Jones just called asking for a medicine. You can figure it out that way.

"A big part of this for me is dealing with the customers. If you like to talk to people, you'll find this work very satisfying. It's the reason I went into it, you get to meet a lot of interesting people. It's almost like the old fashioned barber shop, you know what's going on, you're a part of the community."

How Frank Maluda Got Started

"In high school I was science-oriented. It was either going to be oceanography or pharmacy. But among other things, I realized oceanography wasn't going to be as flexible as pharmacy. You can be a pharmacist anywhere; but you can't go to Oklahoma and say 'Hey, I'm an oceanographer, give me a job.' One year into community college I decided. I graduated from Berkshire Community College in Massachusetts with an A.A. in Environmental Studies, then I studied for a five-year degree—a Bachelor's of Pharmacy—at Massachusetts College of Pharmacy and graduated in 1979.

"It had always been my goal to own my own business. Though things are pretty level now, back then hospital pharmacy was paying less than retail pharmacy.

"I did internships in hospitals and retail stores and I found I enjoyed visiting with customers more in a retail setting than seeing the nurses peek their heads through the window asking for orders. In a retail store, I have more contact with customers."

Expert Advice

"As far as getting off to a good foot, I would recommend going for a sixth year to get your doctorate in pharmacy. If you choose to work in an institutional pharmacy, such as in a hospitals, you'll get a better base pay.

"I've had no regrets as far as the retail end of it, but there is one major problem facing all independents these days. HMOs send all their patients to a particular pharmacy of their choosing. It can leave a lot of independents out in the cold.

"And now it's becoming political. The independents have joined together and there are bills out there to allow us to get into these HMO circles. Otherwise, it seems as if it's coming down to having only two pharmacies in the whole country.

"Because of this, until things get settled, I would encourage someone to consider a hospital setting instead of owning their own business.

"And here's another tip; in pharmacy school you're not given a lot of business courses, but if you are thinking of going the independent route, it would be important to have that business background.

"Finally, I feel it's very important to have sympathy for my customers. They can have cancer or AIDS and sometimes they like to know that there's someone out there who will just listen."

●　　●　　●

FOR MORE INFORMATION

For information on pharmacy as a career, preprofessional and professional requirements, programs offered by all the colleges of pharmacy, and student financial aid, contact:

American Association of Colleges of Pharmacy
1426 Prince Street
Alexandria, VA 22314

Information on requirements for licensure in a particular state is available from the Board of Pharmacy of the state or from:

National Association of Boards of Pharmacy
700 Busse Hwy
Park Ridge, IL 60068

Information on careers with pharmaceutical companies is available from:

American Pharmaceutical Association
2215 Constitution Avenue, NW
Washington, DC 20037-2985

CHAPTER 13 Veterinarians

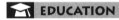

EDUCATION
Post Graduate Required

$$$ SALARY/EARNINGS
$20,000 to $75,000

OVERVIEW

Veterinarians examine, diagnose, and treat animals for any type of medical problem. While some have a general practice treating all kinds of animals, most work with either small pets or with large animals such as horses, swine, sheep, and cattle. Veterinarians also advise owners on the care and breeding of their animals.

Veterinary Specialists

Just as medical doctors have areas of specialization, so do veterinarians. Although most go into general practice, others specialize in, for example, veterinary ophthalmology, cardiology, orthopedics, or specialized surgery.

Relief Veterinarians

Relief veterinarians function much as substitute teachers do. They work for different practices on an on-call basis, filling in for vacationing vets or during emergencies. They're usually paid for the day, with earnings varying from $150 to $300, depending on how much experience they have and the area of the country in which they practice.

Research and Food Safety Inspection

Veterinarians contribute to human as well as animal health. Some vets engage in research to prevent and treat diseases in humans. They also help prevent the outbreak of rabies or other diseases that can be transmitted to humans and may quarantine animals or perform autopsies when necessary.

Veterinarians who are meat inspectors examine slaughtering and processing plants, check live animals and carcasses for disease, and enforce government food purity and sanitation regulations.

JOB SETTINGS

Most vets work in animal clinics or hospitals, but some also work for the government, public health, universities, zoos, and race tracks. Relief veterinarians have a variety of offices for which they work and vets can also choose to travel further afield, wherever their services are needed.

TRAINING

All vets must be licensed, and to become licensed, vets must have a Doctor of Veterinary Medicine degree (D.V.M. or V.M.D.) from an accredited college of veterinary medicine and pass a state board exam.

For research and/or teaching positions, a master's or Ph.D. is usually required. For a specialty certification a veterinarian must complete a three-year residency program and pass an examination.

The D.V.M. degree requires a minimum of six years of college, two of preveterinary study (physical and biological sciences) and four years of vet school. But because admission to a school of veterinary medicine is very competitive, most successful applicants have completed four years of undergraduate work before they apply.

SALARIES

According to the American Veterinary Medical Association, the average starting salary of 1991 veterinary medical college graduates was $27,858. The average income of veterinarians in private practice was $63,069.

The average annual salary for veterinarians in the federal government in nonsupervisory, supervisory, and managerial positions was $50,482 in 1993.

EDUCATION
H.S. Required
On-the-Job Training Possible
A.A./A.S. Recommended

$$$ SALARY/EARNINGS
Minimum Wage to $20,000

VETERINARIAN ASSISTANTS AND TECHNICIANS

Just as medical doctors rely heavily on nurses and other medical personnel, so do veterinarians depend on assistants and technicians. These workers are a valuable asset to any practice.

Some assistants (also called kennel workers) and technicians are successful landing a job without formal training and are taught the skills they need on the job. However, many vets these days require their technicians to have gone through a formal training program. (The address for information on education for vet techs is listed at the end of this chapter.) In addition, a vet tech can expect his or her salary to increase with an official diploma or certificate.

RELATED FIELDS

Other occupations that involve working with animals include animal trainers, zoologists, marine biologists, and naturalists.

INTERVIEW

Lance Weidenbaum
Veterinarian

Dr. Lance Weidenbaum owns the Deer Run Animal Hospital, a small pet clinic, in Deerfield Beach, Florida. He is entitled to use the designation D.V.M. (Doctor of Veterinary Medicine) after his name.

What the Job's Really Like

"My days really differ one day to another. As a small animal practice owner I do not only veterinary work, but managerial work. So for instance, in a day I might do three or four surgeries. Some of them will be straightforward, like spays or neuters, sometimes there'll be a laceration or a wound. I'll see some appointments in the exam rooms and treat various things such as ear infections, skin problems, or diarrhea. I may do some vaccines. The other part of the day I have paperwork to do. I'll review records, go over invoices, handle a range of phone calls, back paperwork, ordering supplies, that sort of thing. Before you know it the day is over.

"It never really gets boring, there's always so many different things to do. The thing that makes it exciting is that occasionally we'll see an unusual case or an animal that's in serious condition, that we can make better.

"But that excitement doesn't always happen. Sometimes you won't see anything other than flea or skin problems. That can get humdrum, especially in South Florida where we have a huge flea problem.

"At my clinic I don't see that many trauma cases, trauma cases being animals hit by cars or injured in dog fights. In the area where I am most people keep their animals inside. We're not a St. Elsewhere/ER type of place. Although trauma, of course, isn't good for the animals, from a professional standpoint it's exciting seeing all that kind of stuff going on.

"I mainly treat dogs and cats, occasionally hamsters or gerbils or rabbits. Very infrequently I'll see some birds, but anything serious I'd send to a specialist. I do utilize specialists, if there's something beyond my expertise. A few weeks ago we had a dog who broke his thigh bone in half and needed a plate. We had a specialist come in to do the operation.

"And sometimes the animals we see are difficult to deal with. Just today we had a cat come in with an infection, but we couldn't even look at it because he was too upset. We had to give him a tranquilizer and then when he'd calmed down enough, we were able to take a look at it and treat it.

"There are some hazards, too. If you're not careful you can get bitten, you can get scratched, but if you exercise caution it doesn't really happen that often. You can't trust every animal, especially when they're in a setting where nice things aren't going to happen to them. They're going to be injected and prodded and poked, and their natural impulse may be to fight back. They don't know they're being helped.

"A downside to the job is that being a practice owner, if it's slow, you worry about business. And you have problems that are not exclusive to being a veterinarian. They can happen in any business. For example, you have to deal with personnel or clients not paying their bills. Or sometimes you get clients that no matter what you do or how well you take care of their animals, they find fault. Thank goodness that's few and far between.

"The upsides are working up a complex case and being able to save the animal. That's a real positive bonus. The other thing is being a business owner, even though I work a lot, I have a lot of independence. If I want to go out for an hour or two, unless I have people waiting for me, I can go. I'm not responsible to anybody. But if you're an employee, you only have certain times when you can leave. It provides a good income, a good quality of life and I enjoy running a practice and the independence it gives me.

"Earnings really vary, though. Veterinarians are grossly underpaid. If you look at the training we go through; we have to go through four years of college and then another four years of medical school. And, often, the veterinarian doctor that comes out owes $30,000 to $50,000 in school loans. The beginning graduates coming out nowadays are earning only between $28,000 and $32,000 a year as an employee of an existing practice. Bus drivers probably make that much. MDs come out and command 75 to 100 grand. Business owners themselves can make $50,000, then there's some–maybe race horse vets–who can make a million. But that's not common. Some vets, though, can do quite well, they own three or four or five practices. And an employee vet with experience can make between $30,000 to $70,000.

"But don't forget, the business owner also has a major outlay for equipment and such. When I started my place, I had a business loan, which I paid back. You're behind the eight ball for a while. It can take a long time to get out of the hole."

How Lance Weidenbaum Got Started

"A lot of my colleagues and friends all knew they wanted to be vets since they were four or five. They grew up on farms and used to see the vet come out and knew that's what they wanted to do. I grew up in Brooklyn, New York and you don't see many vets coming out there. So I really didn't have an early interest. I took a break from college when I was around 19 or 20 and, this was a time when you were able to do this, I hitchhiked around North America and I took my dog with me. We were hitching across Canada and late one night I got a ride from someone who had bought some Kentucky Fried Chicken and gave it to my dog without my knowledge. She started choking. We went to an emergency place and had a vet come out to meet us at about midnight. He was able to treat her and she was fine, but I told him I really didn't have much money. He said to me that this one was on him and that maybe one day I'd repay it in some way. I loved the way he worked and the experience gave me a spark. I decided to go back to school and I took a lot of science courses and worked real hard at it. I graduated in 1974 from State University New York, New Paltz. Then I went for doctoral work at the University of Minnesota in Minneapolis and after I was there a year, I got accepted into their veterinarian school.

"I worked for three different vets for four or five years and then started my own practice in 1985. I have three other employees, a veterinary technician, a veterinary technician/receptionist, and another receptionist up front. And occasionally I'll have a relief veterinarian come in to spell me."

Expert Advice

"If someone is interested in working with large animals I would suggest they volunteer some time on a farm. If they're interested in small animals, then they should volunteer or even work at a small animal veterinary practice. See if it's all that it's cracked up to be. A lot of times people look at veterinarians and think 'oh, what a glamorous, fun job,' but it's not always like that.

"They should also look into the financial aspects. I was naive when I started. They're going to be borrowing a lot of money and it's going to be tough for the first few years.

"But if all that seems okay, I think it's a great profession. I love it. The bottom line is that you're going to be working for most of your life–why not have a job you like and can make a good living with? I think being a veterinarian affords that."

♦ ♦ ♦

FOR MORE INFORMATION

For information on careers in veterinary medicine and veterinary technology contact:

> American Veterinary Medical Association
> 1931 N. Meacham Rd., Suite 100
> Schaumburg, IL 60173-4360

For information on veterinary education contact:

> Association of American Veterinary Medical Colleges
> 1101 Vermont Ave. NW, Suite 710
> Washington, DC 20005

For information on scholarships, grants, and loans, contact the financial aid office at the veterinary schools to which you wish to apply.

VGM CAREER BOOKS

BUSINESS PORTRAITS
Boeing
Coca-Cola
Ford
McDonald's

CAREER DIRECTORIES
Careers Encyclopedia
Dictionary of Occupational Titles
Occupational Outlook Handbook

CAREERS FOR
Animal Lovers; Bookworms; Caring
People; Computer Buffs; Crafty
People; Culture Lovers;
Environmental Types; Fashion Plates;
Film Buffs; Foreign Language
Aficionados; Good Samaritans;
Gourmets; Health Nuts; History
Buffs; Kids at Heart; Music Lovers;
Mystery Buffs; Nature Lovers; Night
Owls; Number Crunchers; Plant
Lovers; Shutterbugs; Sports Nuts;
Travel Buffs; Writers

CAREERS IN
Accounting; Advertising; Business;
Child Care; Communications;
Computers; Education; Engineering;
the Environment; Finance;
Government; Health Care; High
Tech; Horticulture & Botany;
International Business; Journalism;
Law; Marketing; Medicine; Science;
Social & Rehabilitation Services

CAREER PLANNING
Beating Job Burnout
Beginning Entrepreneur
Big Book of Jobs
Career Planning & Development for
    College Students &
    Recent Graduates
Career Change
Career Success for People with
    Physical Disabilities
Careers Checklists
College and Career Success for Students
    with Learning Disabilities
Complete Guide to Career Etiquette
Cover Letters They Don't Forget
Dr. Job's Complete Career Guide
Executive Job Search Strategies
Guide to Basic Cover Letter Writing
Guide to Basic Résumé Writing
Guide to Internet Job Searching
Guide to Temporary Employment
Job Interviewing for College Students
Joyce Lain Kennedy's Career Book

Out of Uniform
Parent's Crash Course in Career
    Planning
Slame Dunk Résumés
Up Your Grades: Proven Strategies
    for Academic Success

CAREER PORTRAITS
Animals; Cars; Computers;
Electronics; Fashion; Firefighting;
Music; Nature; Nursing; Science;
Sports; Teaching; Travel; Writing

GREAT JOBS FOR
Business Majors
Communications Majors
Engineering Majors
English Majors
Foreign Language Majors
History Majors
Psychology Majors
Sociology Majors

HOW TO
Apply to American Colleges and
    Universities
Approach an Advertising Agency and
    Walk Away with the Job You Want
Be a Super Sitter
Bounce Back Quickly After
    Losing Your Job
Change Your Career
Choose the Right Career
Cómo escribir un currículum vitae en
    inglés que tenga éxito
Find Your New Career Upon
    Retirement
Get & Keep Your First Job
Get Hired Today
Get into the Right Business School
Get into the Right Law School
Get into the Right Medical School
Get People to Do Things Your Way
Have a Winning Job Interview
Hit the Ground Running in Your
    New Job
Hold It All Together When You've
    Lost Your Job
Improve Your Study Skills
Jumpstart a Stalled Career
Land a Better Job
Launch Your Career in TV News
Make the Right Career Moves
Market Your College Degree
Move from College into a
    Secure Job
Negotiate the Raise You Deserve
Prepare Your Curriculum Vitae

Prepare for College
Run Your Own Home Business
Succeed in Advertising When all You
Succeed in College
Succeed in High School
Take Charge of Your Child's Early
    Education
Write a Winning Résumé
Write Successful Cover Letters
Write Term Papers & Reports
Write Your College Application Essay

MADE EASY
College Applications
Cover Letters
Getting a Raise
Job Hunting
Job Interviews
Résumés

**ON THE JOB: REAL PEOPLE
    WORKING IN...**
Communications
Health Care
Sales & Marketing
Service Businesses

OPPORTUNITIES IN
This extensive series provides detailed
    information on more than 150
    individual career fields.

RÉSUMÉS FOR
Advertising Careers
Architecture and Related Careers
Banking and Financial Careers
Business Management Careers
College Students &
    Recent Graduates
Communications Careers
Computer Careers
Education Careers
Engineering Careers
Environmental Careers
Ex-Military Personnel
50+ Job Hunters
Government Careers
Health and Medical Careers
High School Graduates
High Tech Careers
Law Careers
Midcareer Job Changes
Nursing Careers
Re-Entering the Job Market
Sales and Marketing Careers
Scientific and Technical Careers
Social Service Careers
The First-Time Job Hunter

 VGM Career Horizons
a division of *NTC Publishing Group*
4255 West Touhy Avenue
Lincolnwood, Illinois 60646–1975

MAY 3 0 1997